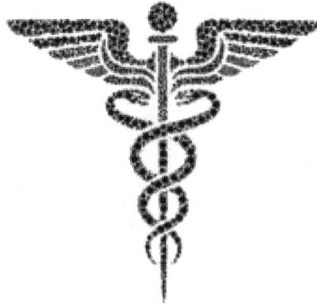

ALZHEIMER'S
& OTHER DEMENTIAS:

A Caregiver's Guide

BY
DR. ANNETTE ACEVEDO HERNANDEZ, MD, CDS
Collaboration by DR. GILFREDY ACEVEDO HERNANDEZ, MD
Translation by CAMILLE A. SCHWINGHAMMER, MSMS

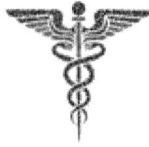

COPYRIGHT

Copyright © 2024 by Dr. Annette Acevedo Hernandez
Printed in Colombia
Linotipia Martínez Printing, 2024
ISBN 979-8-9900969-0-5

www.DementiaCareMD.com

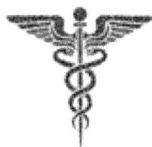

PREFACE

THE MAIN MOTIVATION behind the writing of this book is to share our experience as medical professionals, medical directors of a nursing home for over 20 years, and children of a patient who had Alzheimer's disease to improve the quality of life of those patients and their families.

Over more than 25 years ago, our family was impacted by the sad news that our father had Alzheimer's. For us, as his children, the diagnosis was devastating. Still, for our mother, the situation was more complex as she faced not only the pain of the diagnosis of her beloved husband, but the challenge of being the caregiver of a patient with Alzheimer's. All without the knowledge or preparation to be able to offer excellent care, only the love she felt for her husband.

These experiences, combined with the alarming figures reported to date that place Alzheimer's and other dementias as the sixth cause of death in the U.S. and the seventh cause of death in the world, impact and awaken the social responsibility to educate and guide others to diminish the fear, frustration, and anxiety caused by the diagnosis of Alzheimer's and other dementias.

This guide has the objective of offering guidance to caregivers, health professionals, family, and friends of patients with Alzheimer's or other dementias to improve the quality of life of the patients and their caregivers.

This guide DOES NOT SUBSTITUTE the medical recommendations of your primary care physician, psychiatrist, neurologist, or healthcare team.

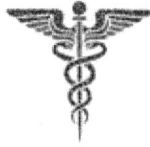

TABLE OF CONTENTS

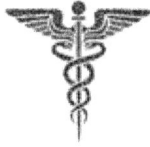

DEDICATION

THIS BOOK is dedicated to our parents, Gilfredy and Gladys. Their love, dedication, and guidance have been the cornerstone of our development, shaping us into the individuals we are today, even in the face of adversity.

To all the families with a loved one diagnosed with Alzheimer's or other dementias, this book is also dedicated to you. May it serve as a source of support, guidance, and understanding as you navigate the challenges of caregiving and strive to provide the best possible care for your loved ones.

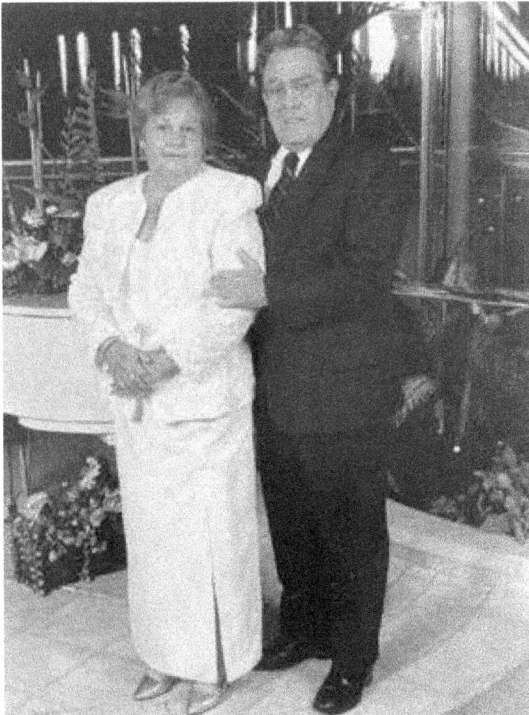

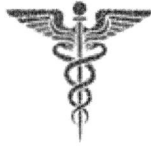

PROLOGUE

1 CORINTHIANS 13:13

So now **Faith, Hope,** and **Love** abide, these three; but the greatest of these is **Love**.

1 CORINTHIANS 13:4-7

"Love is patient and kind; love does not envy or boast; it is not arrogant or rude. It does not insist on its own way; it is not irritable or resentful; it does not rejoice at wrongdoing, but rejoices with the truth. Love bears all things, believes all things, hopes all things, endures all things."

THE LOVE you feel for that loved one is what will guide and help you offer the best care for that patient diagnosed with Alzheimer's or other dementias.

Life is a journey; what's important is to live that journey to the fullest; that is the beauty of life.

Enjoy *more*
Live *more*
Love *more*
Forgive *more*
Help *more*
Share *more*
Be *more* grateful...

So that at the end of your journey, you haven't missed what's most important—the essence of life!

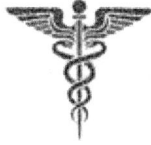

CHAPTER ONE

Alzheimer's Overview

I. INTRODUCTION

ALZHEIMER'S IS a neurodegenerative disease that affects the brains of those diagnosed. The disease progresses slowly, producing significant mental and physical deterioration that interferes with the patient's ability to continue their daily activities, disabling them.

This disease was discovered in 1906, over a century ago, thanks to Dr. Alois Alzheimer, and to this day, while multiple scientific research studies have been conducted, a cure has not been found. However, research has generated important information about the diagnosis, treatment, and leading role that prevention plays in this disease.

In the following few pages, we will review different concepts, statistics, future predictions, treatments, and other aspects to better understand the changes a patient with Alzheimer's experiences. This will help in facing the problem and improving the quality of life for patients with Alzheimer's or other dementias and their families.

II. HISTORY OF ALZHEIMER'S

In 1906, German psychiatrist and neuropathologist Dr. Alois Alzheimer identified the first case of what is now known as Alzheimer's disease. In 1901, Dr. Alzheimer worked as a neuropsychiatrist in a German psychiatric hospital, where he began evaluating a 55-year-old patient admitted to the hospital for memory disturbances, agitation, and paranoia.[1] Dr. Alzheimer evaluated and began treating the woman when he recognized that the symptoms she presented were not associated with any previously identified in other patients with mental disorders.

The doctor continued treating the patient, and when she passed, he requested an autopsy. The autopsy was performed, revealing that the patient's brain was anatomically smaller than the brains of other patients diagnosed with mental disorders. In this way, Dr. Alzheimer discovered the first anatomical change in the brain under the microscope, which is why the disease is named after him.

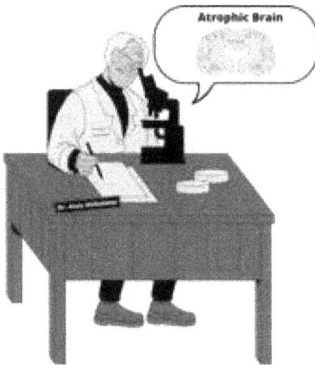

From 1906 until the present, multiple research studies have been conducted to find a cure. Unfortunately, a cure has not been found; however, research has uncovered important information about its prevention, diagnosis, and treatment, offering information that may reduce the prevalence of this disease.

In the following pages, we will review these concepts.

III. WHAT IS ALZHEIMER'S?

Alzheimer's disease is a progressive neurodegenerative syndrome characterized by the loss of behavioral, neurological, and cognitive functions. Some examples of the areas affected by the loss of these functions include:

- ✓ Perception
- ✓ Memory
- ✓ Learning
- ✓ Attention
- ✓ Emotions
- ✓ Social behavior
- ✓ Reasoning
- ✓ Judgment
- ✓ Intelligence
- ✓ Languages

Seventy percent of dementias are caused by Alzheimer's disease. The disease progresses slowly, causing a cognitive decline that weakens mental faculties and interferes with daily activities until eventually causing complete incapacitation. To understand what Alzheimer's is, it is essential to describe the organ affected by this disease—the brain—and its normal functioning in unaffected individuals.

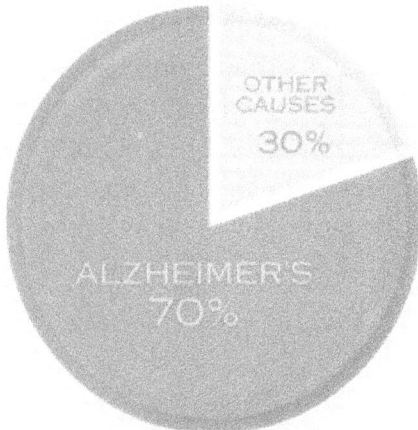

OTHER CAUSES 30%

ALZHEIMER'S 70%

i. *Anatomy of a Healthy Brain*

The brain, anatomically the most complex organ in the human body, weighs approximately 3 pounds (1.36 kg) and is unique in every individual. It is responsible for receiving stimuli through the senses, processing, organizing, and responding to information, it consists of two parts: the left and right hemispheres, each further divided into four lobes. Each lobe specializes in a specific area.

✓ **Temporal Lobe:** Processes information from sensory, auditory, and visual areas. The hippocampus is found in this lobe, the area responsible for memory processing. This area is scientifically identified as the first affected by Alzheimer's disease, which is why patients suffering from this illness present with memory loss.[2] This lobe is also responsible for storing memories of music, which, curiously, are the last memories that these patients tend to forget. This explains why bedridden patients sing their favorite songs but cannot longer swallow.

✓ **Occipital Lobe:** Located in the rear portion of the skull, it receives sensory signals from the eyes. Its functions include the processing and interpretation of vision, allowing for the formation of visual memories.

✓ **Parietal Lobe**: Is found below the parietal bone in the mediolateral portion of the head. Its functions include the perception of tactile stimuli, pressure, temperature, and pain. Perception is the cognitive function that helps us receive, interpret, and comprehend our sensations. Different types of perception exist: visual, tactile, auditory, olfactory, gustative, and temporal movement, among others.

✓ **Frontal Lobe:** This is the biggest lobe of the brain and is found in the frontal section of the skull. Its functions include processing taste, tact, movement, and temperature information. In most people, the left frontal lobe controls language, while the right frontal lobe controls nonverbal signals, such as facial expressions.

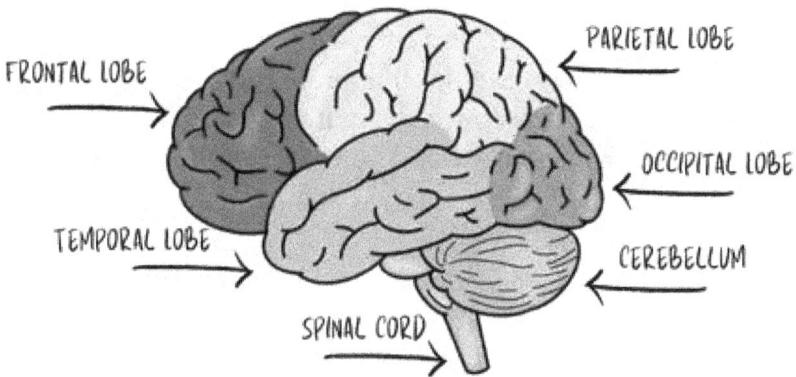

FRONTAL LOBE

PARIETAL LOBE

OCCIPITAL LOBE

TEMPORAL LOBE

CEREBELLUM

SPINAL CORD

ii. Function of a Healthy Brain

The brain plays a fundamental role in ensuring survival and overseeing vital functions such as coordination, balance, language, and memory. Its intricate operations are governed by millions of nerve cells known as neurons. These neurons interact by receiving stimuli and communicating with one another through a process called synapsis. This intricate form of communication, facilitated by neurotransmitters, enables the exchange of nutrients between neurons and the processing of stimuli essential for proper brain function.

Chemical neurotransmitter, also called *"chemical mediators,"* are crucial in facilitating communication between cells within the brain. These mediators must be present in specific proportions to ensure the brain operates effectively. Neurons receive input from sensory organs, capture information from the external world, and transmit responses to various parts of the body through the nervous system.

Essentially, the brain acts as the command center for our body's functions, orchestrating a complex interplay of neurons and chemical messengers to interpret sensory input and coordinate responses. Understanding these mechanisms sheds light on the intricate workings of the brain and underscores the importance of maintaining its delicate balance for overall well-being and functioning.

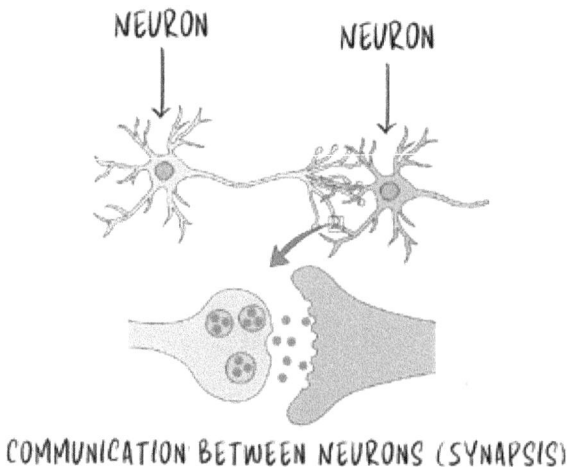

NEURON   NEURON

COMMUNICATION BETWEEN NEURONS (SYNAPSIS)

iii. Brain Anatomy of an Alzheimer's Patient

In Alzheimer's disease, the brain undergoes a reduction in size and weight due to the death of neurons. Tau proteins and beta-amyloid pro-teins may become toxic, causing neuron degeneration when present in abnormal proportions.[2] This disproportionate accumulation can also interrupt synapses, inhibiting nutrients from reaching neurons and causing their death while disrupting the stimulus-response. Due to the death of these neurons, the brain becomes smaller and atrophied; this was Dr. Alois Alzheimer's first discovery.

Alzheimer's disease research holds a crucial position worldwide because of its significant impact on both economic and social aspects. The United States government has even promoted the creation of a project titled NAPA (National Alzheimer's Project Act), which aims to advance research studies to find a cure and develop strategies to assist Alzheimer's patients and their families. This project has been active since 2011 and was unanimously approved by the U.S. government; CMS "Clinical Medical Services" (the U.S. agency in charge of fulfilling the NAPA law) annually presents a report that includes recommendations for improving the quality of life for patients diagnosed with Alzheimer's and other dementias.[3]

It is important to clarify that alterations in cognitive areas and dementia are not part of normal aging. The aging process typically involves decreased and slowed thinking, reasoning, and learning, but not dementia.

IV. DIFFERENCES BETWEEN ALZHEIMER'S AND DEMENTIA

Alzheimer's and dementia are not the same. Dementia is a syndrome or a set of signs and symptoms that manifest with cognitive impairment, interfering with the patient's daily activities and thereby incapacitating them.[4] Alzheimer's is one of the leading causes of dementia, and according to the World Health Organization (WHO), it accounts for sixty to seventy percent of dementia cases.[5] Additionally, dementia may arise from other causes, including reversible and irreversible forms.

i. **Reversible Dementias:** Reversible dementias are those in which the brain has the potential to recover, and the patient is left without cognitive impairment once the disease is cured. It's important to note that while some dementias caused by reversible factors can be fully resolved with treatment, others may only partially improve or may leave some residual cognitive impairment. Additionally, prompt diagnosis and intervention are crucial for maximizing the chances of recovery in cases of reversible dementia. Therefore, thorough medical evaluation and appropriate diagnostic testing are essential for identifying and addressing potentially reversible causes of cognitive impairment. Some examples of this subtype of dementia include:

    ✓ **Depression:** Depression can mimic symptoms of dementia, such as memory problems, cognitive difficulties, and changes in behavior. However, unlike irreversible dementias, treating depression with therapy, medication, or a combination of both can often lead to significant improvement or resolution of cognitive symptoms.

    ✓ **Drug Use:** Substance abuse, including alcohol abuse, can cause cognitive impairment that may resemble dementia. With appropriate treatment and cessation of drug use, cognitive function may improve, although recovery may vary depending on factors such as the severity and duration of substance abuse.

✓ **Tumors:** Dementia symptoms caused by brain tumors may be reversible if the tumor is successfully treated or removed. Once the tumor is addressed, cognitive function may improve, although recovery can depend on factors such as the size, location, and malignancy of the tumor.

✓ **Vitamin Deficiencies:** Certain vitamin deficiencies, such as deficiencies in vitamin B12, thiamine (vitamin B1), or niacin (vitamin B3), can lead to cognitive impairment that may be reversible with adequate supplementation or dietary changes. Treating the underlying deficiency can help restore cognitive function in some cases.

✓ **Metabolic Disorders**: Metabolic diseases like Addison's disease or Cushing's disease can present with cognitive impairment symptoms due to disruptions in hormonal balance or electrolyte levels. These symptoms may include confusion, memory problems, and difficulty concentrating. Prompt diagnosis and management of the underlying metabolic condition can often lead to the resolution of cognitive symptoms, highlighting the importance of thorough medical evaluation in cases of cognitive decline.

✓ **Anesthesia Complications**: Certain medications administered during general anesthesia, particularly in older adults or individuals with pre-existing cognitive vulnerabilities, may cause cognitive side effects postoperatively. These effects can range from temporary confusion to more persistent cognitive deficits. Factors such as the type and dosage of anesthesia, duration of exposure, and individual susceptibility can influence the severity and duration of these complications. Vigilant monitoring and appropriate postoperative care are essential to mitigate these risks and support cognitive recovery.

✓**Others:** Other reversible causes of dementia may include thyroid dysfunction, infections (such as urinary tract infections or meningitis), and adverse drug reactions. Identifying and treating the underlying cause can often lead to improvement or resolution of cognitive symptoms.

ii. *Irreversible Dementias:* Irreversible dementias are those that leave patients with permanent damage to the brain. Each of these irreversible dementias presents unique challenges for caregivers and requires tailored approaches to care and management. Understanding the specific symptoms and progression of each condition can help caregivers provide support and assistance to individuals affected by dementia. Examples include:

✓ **Alzheimer's Disease:** Alzheimer's is the most common form of irreversible dementia, characterized by progressive memory loss, cognitive decline, and changes in behavior and personality. It involves the accumulation of abnormal protein deposits in the brain.

✓ **Lewy Body Dementia (LBD):** LBD is a type of dementia associated with abnormal protein deposits called Lewy bodies in the brain. Symptoms may include visual hallucinations, fluctuations in alertness, tremors, and problems with movement.

✓ **Parkinson's Disease:** Parkinson's disease is a neurodegenerative disorder characterized by the progressive loss of neurons, leading to motor impairments such as tremors, bradykinesia, and postural instability, alongside cognitive alterations. These cognitive changes can manifest as difficulties in executive function, attention, and visuospatial abilities, often impacting daily functioning.

✓ **Tumors:** Depending on their type and location (benign or malignant), brain tumors can produce dementia-like symptoms, including memory impairment, reasoning difficulties, bradykinesia, rigidity, and speech disturbances. The extent of cognitive impairment can vary, and in some cases, may be irreversible.

✓ **Mild Cognitive Impairment (MCI):** MCI manifests as subtle cognitive changes, such as forgetfulness, difficulty in remembering recent events or conversations, and challenges with decision-making or problem-solving. These symptoms, while noticeable, do not significantly impair daily functioning and are often early indicators of potential progression to Alzheimer's disease or other forms of dementia.

✓ **Frontotemporal Dementia (FTD):** FTD encompasses a group of disorders characterized by progressive damage to the frontal and temporal lobes of the brain. Symptoms may include changes in behavior, personality, language difficulties, and problems with executive functions.

> ➤ **Pick's Disease:** Pick's disease, a rare form of frontotemporal dementia, is characterized by abnormal accumulation of Pick bodies in specific areas of the brain. Common symptoms include compulsive behaviors, social disinhibition, language difficulties, and apathy. This subtype of dementia typically presents with prominent behavioral and personality changes in contrast to memory impairment seen in Alzheimer's disease.

✓ **Creutzfeldt-Jakob Disease (CJD):** CJD is a rare and rapidly progressive neurological disorder caused by abnormal prion proteins. Symptoms may include involuntary movements, coordination difficulties, cognitive decline, and memory disturbances. The disease has a rapid clinical course, often resulting in severe neurological impairment and death within months to a few years of onset.

✓ **Huntington's disease:** Huntington's disease is an inheritable neurodegenerative disorder marked by motor abnormalities, psychiatric disturbances, and cognitive deterioration. It results from a mutation in the huntingtin gene, leading to the accumulation of abnormal proteins in the brain. This condition profoundly impacts individuals' quality of life, necessitating comprehensive care and support strategies.

✓ **Vascular Dementia:** Vascular dementia results from impaired blood flow to the brain, often due to cerebrovascular accidents or the accumulation of abnormal plaques. Symptoms can vary depending on the location and extent of the vascular damage and may resemble those of other forms of dementia, including memory disturbances, judgment impairments, and executive dysfunction.

In conclusion, distinguishing between reversible and irreversible dementias is paramount in understanding the prognosis and management of cognitive impairment. While irreversible dementias, such as Alzheimer's disease and frontotemporal dementia, entail progressive neurodegenerative processes resulting in permanent cognitive decline, reversible dementias offer hope for recovery through targeted interventions. Addressing underlying causes such as depression, substance abuse, tumors, and vitamin deficiencies can lead to significant improvements in cognitive function. Making an early diagnosis is crucial to the correct treatment of the patient and can help prevent fear, frustration, and disorientation for both the patient and their family.

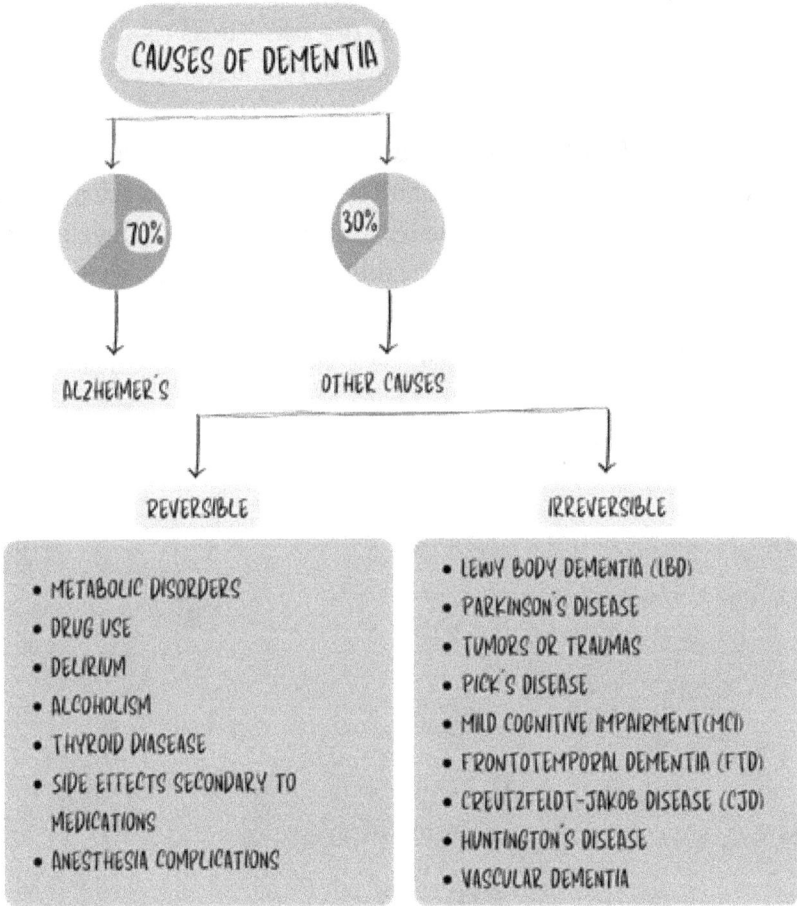

V. CAUSES OF ALZHEIMER'S

Alzheimer's is a neurodegenerative brain disease; the exact cause of this disease is unknown. Thanks to research, some risk factors may increase the possibility of developing this disease. These risk factors can be divided into modifiable and non-modifiable risk factors.

i. **Non-Modifiable Risk Factors:** Non-modifiable risk factors cannot be changed, varied, or altered; these factors are age and genetics. Age is considered the leading risk factor for developing this disease. Genetically speaking, the APOE-4 gene increases the risk of developing this disease, but its presence alone is not enough to cause Alzheimer's. That's why this disease is not classified as a hereditary disease.

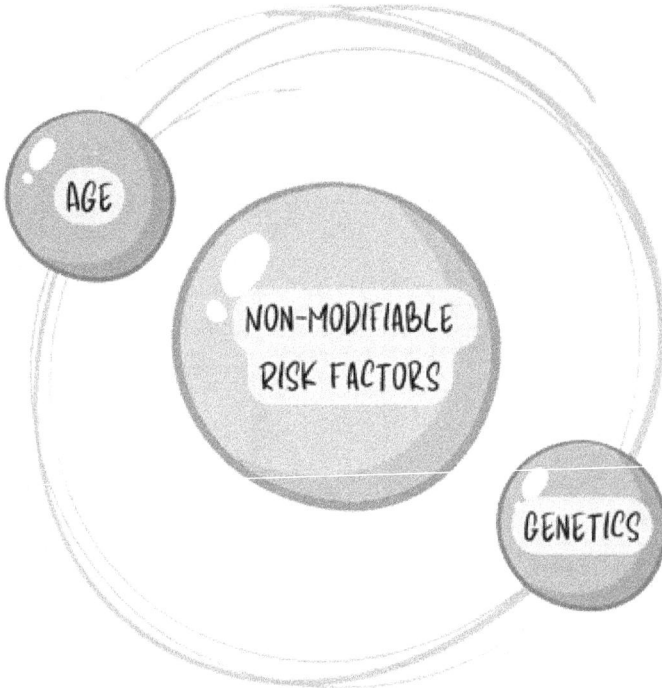

ii. *Modifiable Risk Factors:* Modifiable risk factors, along with lifestyle changes, may decrease the risk of developing Alzheimer's disease. These risk factors include a sedentary lifestyle, smoking, hypertension, depression, Type II diabetes, obesity, hyperlipidemia, stress, insomnia, anxiety, a poor diet, and isolation, among others.

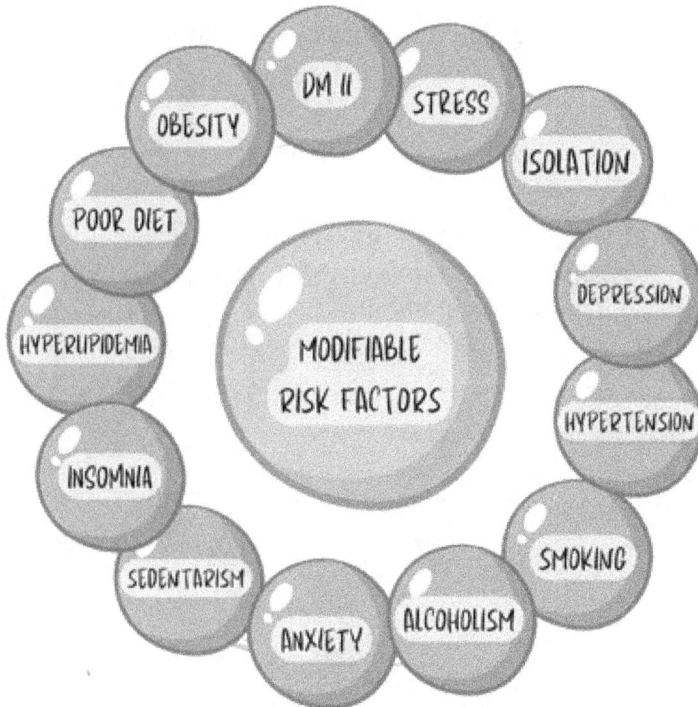

Focusing on modifiable factors and making lifestyle changes to reduce the likelihood of developing Alzheimer's disease is crucial. We should never dwell on the risks of family members developing Alzheimer's, as the stress and anxiety caused by such concerns could be a triggering factor for the development of this disease.

VI. SYMPTOMS

Alzheimer's is a progressive neurodegenerative disease that initially affects memory. The symptomatology of this disease varies from patient to patient, owing to the diversity in its progression, duration, and chronology of its symptoms. Research into this disease has concluded that the initial anatomical changes in the brain appear years before patients display the first symptoms.[6] These symptoms include cognitive and non-cognitive alterations, as well as physical changes.

Non-cognitive symptoms consist of behavioral and psychiatric changes that could be confused with other mental illnesses. While physical symptoms consist of physiological alterations such as changes in gait, motor function, and sensory perception, reflecting the multifaceted nature of Alzheimer's disease progression.

i. *Cognitive Symptoms*

- ✓ Memory alterations
- ✓ Difficulty speaking
- ✓ Difficulty reasoning
- ✓ Lack of judgment
- ✓ Learning problems

ii. *Non-Cognitive Symptoms* [7]

- ✓ Delusions
- ✓ Irritability
- ✓ Anxiety
- ✓ Frustration
- ✓ Aggression
- ✓ Agitation
- ✓ Apathy
- ✓ Depression
- ✓ Disorientation in place, time, and person

✓ Behavioral and personality changes
✓ Directionless wandering
✓ Repetitive screaming
✓ Sexual disinhibition
✓ Psychosis
✓ Sleep Disturbances

iii. *Physical Symptoms*

✓ Difficulty walking
✓ Loss of balance
✓ Problems swallowing
✓ Incontinence problems
✓ Joint stiffness
✓ Major Fatigue
✓ Muscular and extremity weakness
✓ Muscle Mass Loss
✓ Pressure ulcers
✓ Symptoms secondary to infectious processes
✓ Symptoms related to chronic conditions

It is essential to educate ourselves and understand that the symptomatology of this disease varies for each patient. Consequently, the treatment for each patient is different. This is why we should avoid comparisons between treatments to prevent confusion. The treatment for each patient with Alzheimer's is individualized and directed toward the patient's unique presentation of symptoms.

VII: DIAGNOSIS

Alzheimer's disease cannot be diagnosed through a laboratory test or radiology imaging. A definitive diagnosis can only be given once the patient has died, via autopsy. However, thanks to research, there are tools available that can help us diagnose Alzheimer's with almost 90% accuracy. The most important thing to keep in mind when considering a diagnosis is to try to visit a healthcare professional who can make a diagnosis as soon as possible in order to start the patient on a tailored treatment plan. The evaluation of a patient consists of:

i. *Clinical Exam*

- ✓ **Medical History:** The patient's medical history will provide all of their information up to the point of evaluation, including illnesses, past history, present medications, previous results, and signs & symptoms that they may present at the time of assessment.

- ✓ **Physical Exam:** The healthcare provider will examine the patient's physical state to determine if any physical problems exist. The provider will examine, auscultate, explore, and palpate their body.

- ✓ **Visual Exam:** Visual impairments may be related to Alzheimer's disease, which is why a visual exam is important when evaluating a patient with dementia.

- ✓ **Dental Exam:** Dental exams are crucial every six months due to emerging research suggesting a link between certain bacteria (currently under investigation) and an increased risk of developing Alzheimer's.[8]

- ✓ **Auditory Exam:** The auditory exam is essential, as certain findings could indicate an elevated risk of developing Alzheimer's.

ii. ***Laboratory Tests:*** To identify some potential alterations, the following laboratory tests should be conducted:

- ✓ **CBC (Complete Blood Count):** A CBC test measures various components of the blood, including red blood cells, white blood cells, and platelets. While it doesn't directly diagnose Alzheimer's, it helps rule out other conditions that could contribute to cognitive impairment, such as infections or anemia.

- ✓ **UA (Urinalysis):** A Urinalysis evaluates urine's physical and chemical properties. It can help identify urinary tract infections or kidney problems, which may present symptoms similar to Alzheimer's or exacerbate cognitive decline.

- ✓ **CMP (Comprehensive Metabolic Panel):** A CMP test assesses kidney function, liver function, electrolyte levels, and blood glucose levels. Abnormalities in these parameters could indicate underlying health issues that may affect brain function and contribute to cognitive decline.

- ✓ **VDRL (Venereal Disease Research Laboratory) Test:** The VDRL test is used to screen for syphilis, a sexually transmitted infection. While syphilis is not directly linked to Alzheimer's, untreated syphilis can lead to neurological complications that may mimic symptoms of dementia.

- ✓ **HIV (Human Immunodeficiency Virus) Test:** HIV can affect the central nervous system and lead to cognitive impairment, known as HIV-associated neurocognitive disorders (HAND). Testing for HIV is important to rule out HIV-related causes of cognitive decline.

- ✓ **Vitamin B12 Levels:** Vitamin B12 deficiency can cause neurological symptoms, including cognitive impairment and dementia-like symptoms. Measuring vitamin B12 levels helps identify potential deficiencies contributing to cognitive decline.

✓**TSH (Thyroid-Stimulating Hormone) Test:** Thyroid dysfunction, such as hypothyroidism, can manifest with cognitive symptoms resembling dementia. A TSH test helps assess thyroid function and rule out thyroid-related causes of cognitive impairment.

iii. Biomarker Studies

✓ **LP:** A lumbar puncture or spinal tap is used to help identify beta-amyloid and Tau proteins in the cerebrospinal fluid (CSF). These biomarkers are recognized as diagnostic evidence of Alzheimer's disease.[9]

✓ **MRI:** This magnetic resonance study provides information about the brain's anatomical structure. The initial changes in the temporomedial lobe, affecting memory and learning in these patients, can be observed. Magnetic resonance enables the identification of brain atrophy causing Alzheimer's.

✓ **PET:** Also known as positron emission tomography, these scans detect characteristic brain changes such as amyloid plaques and tau tangles, aiding in accurate diagnosis. Additionally, PET scans can differentiate between different types of dementia and monitor disease progression over time, providing valuable insights for treatment planning.[10]

✓ **CT SCAN:** This is an X-ray and computerized tomography exam which generates cross-sectional images of the brain. [10]

iv. Neuropsychological Exams

✓ **Mental Exam:** Evaluates memory, language, orientation, executive function, etc. This exam lasts around 10 minutes, and it provides a snapshot of the individual's cognitive status.

✓ **MoCA:** Also known as the Montreal Cognitive Assessment, this exam evaluates cognitive function and helps detect early-onset dementia.[11]

✓ **Mini COG:** This exam is a cognitive screening tool that combines memory evaluation with the clock test and can be used to determine dementia in around 3 minutes.

➢**Clock-Drawing Test (CDT):** The clock-drawing test is a cognitive screening tool often used to detect cognitive impairment, including Alzheimer's disease. In this test, individuals are instructed to draw a clock face, including numbers and hands, to indicate a specific time, typically ten past 11. Errors such as missing numbers, incorrect placement of numbers, and inaccuracies in depicting the time requested can indicate difficulties with spatial organization, planning, and executive function, which are commonly associated with Alzheimer's and other forms of dementia. This simple yet effective test provides valuable insights into cognitive abilities and aids in the early identification of potential cognitive decline.

The main objective is to diagnose Alzheimer's as early as possible for patients to be able to start treatment promptly. Unfortunately, in most cases, the diagnosis occurs when the patient already exhibits signs and symptoms, indicating that cognitive impairment has begun. Identifying this disease during its preclinical phase is limited due to the restricted availability and access to tests that determine biomarkers.

A definitive diagnosis is established through autopsy, thanks to research that has facilitated the development of tools for the precise diagnosis of Alzheimer's at that time. The diagnosis of Alzheimer's is primarily carried out by primary care physicians, using clinical exams along with neuropsychological exams. Currently, researchers mainly use the identification of biomarkers.

VIII: TREATMENT

Alzheimer's does not have a cure. Currently, there are pharmacological medications that, when started during the early stages, may slow down cognitive impairment. The treatment for these patients includes both pharmacological therapy and non-pharmacological therapy.

i. ***Pharmacological Therapy:*** Pharmacological therapy used to treat Alzheimer's consists of two types of available medications that have been approved for the treatment of this disease.

  ✓ **Anti-Cholinergic Drugs:** These inhibit anticholinesterase, the enzyme responsible for the destruction of acetylcholine. Acetylcholine is the neurotransmitter responsible for learning, memory, and concentration. In Alzheimer's patients, acetylcholine is decreased. These anticholinergic medications help improve the cognitive aspect of this disease. They should be started as a form of pharmacological therapy as soon as an Alzheimer's diagnosis is made and should be continued until the final stages of the disease. The following are the three available anticholinergic medications on the market:

  ➢ Donepezil
  ➢ Galantamine
  ➢ Rivastigmine

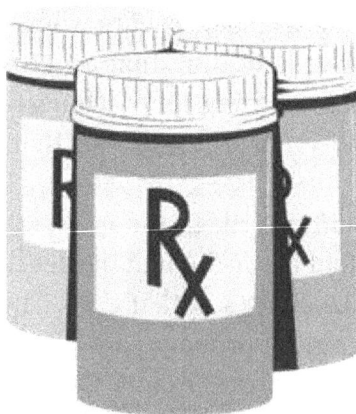

✓ **<u>Glutamate Receptor Antagonist Drugs:</u>** Glutamate is a vital chemical involved in learning and memory, regulated by its controlled release. In patients with neurodegenerative diseases like Alzheimer's, there is an abnormal release of this neurotransmitter. This excess release leads to the degeneration of neurons, resulting in neurodegenerative diseases such as Alzheimer's.

> **Memantine:** is an example of a medication used to regulate glutamate levels.

✓ **<u>Psychiatric Drugs:</u>** In the treatment of Alzheimer's patients, pharmacopsychiatry can be utilized for those experiencing psychiatric symptoms such as depression, apathy, delusions, confusion, hallucinations, aggression, agitation, and disorientation, among others. These symptoms are often part of the cognitive impairment process, and the physician will assess and prescribe medication based on the specific symptoms observed.

ii. *Non-Pharmacological Therapies:* There are non-pharmacological therapies that can potentially enhance the quality of life of Alzheimer's patients. Non-pharmacological treatments encompass interventional therapies that do not involve the use of chemical drugs. Research studies have indicated that combining non-pharmacological treatments with pharmacological treatments may delay cognitive deterioration and reduce behavioral changes, ultimately improving the quality of life for patients and their caregivers. Some examples include: animal therapy[12], music therapy[13], and tai chi[14].

iii. Pharmacological Drugs Being Studied

✓ **Aducanumab:** This medication has received FDA approval for patients with Alzheimer's and MCI. It represents a groundbreaking development as the first drug to target the underlying pathophysiology of the disease. In its early stages, it may slow down the progression of Alzheimer's, emphasizing the critical importance of early diagnosis.[15]However, its current availability is limited, and efforts are underway to have health insurance cover its cost.

✓ **Lecanemab-irmb:** Another medication under study for potential use in Alzheimer's and MCI patients is Leqembi™ (lecanemab-irmb). The primary goal of this medication is to prevent the formation of amyloid plaques and halt cognitive dete-rioration.[16]

In conclusion, it is crucial to educate ourselves and understand that Alzheimer's disease currently lacks a cure. Medications such as Donepezil, Galantamine, Rivastigmine (anticholinergic drugs), and Memantine (an antagonist glutamate receptor medication) do not provide a cure. Instead, these medications delay the onset of non-cognitive, cognitive, and physical symptoms. It's essential to recognize that the treatment for each patient is individualized and should not be compared to that of other individuals who have Alzheimer's or other forms of dementia.

IX: RISK FACTORS

Two categories of risk factors increase the probability of developing Alzheimer's or other dementias: non-modifiable risk factors and modifiable risk factors.

i. **Non-Modifiable Risk Factors:** These factors cannot be controlled or modified, making it essential to focus on the modifiable ones.

   ✓ **Age:** Age plays a primary role among non-modifiable risk factors. The risk increases notably with advancing age, with older individuals facing a significantly heightened susceptibility to the disease.[17] Since aging cannot be prevented, there is nothing that can be done to change this risk factor.

   ✓ **Genetics:** Another pivotal risk factor is the presence of the APOE-4 gene located on chromosome 19, considered a genetic risk factor. While this gene increases the risk of developing Alzheimer's, its presence alone is not indicative of a person developing the disease.[18]

ii. **Modifiable Risk Factors:** These risk factors can be modified or intervened to help avoid, decrease, or control the disease.

   ✓ **Type II DM:** While research is ongoing to explain the relationship between diabetes and dementia, it is established that a diagnosis of type 2 diabetes is a risk factor for developing Alzheimer's. Diabetes is often found in overweight individuals with a lack of exercise, leading to a higher risk of brain strokes, cardiovascular disease, and mental illnesses, all of which are risk factors for Alzheimer's. Physio-pathologically, high sugar levels adversely affect the brain.

   ✓ **Hypertension:** Studies show that patients with high blood pressure are at a higher risk of being diagnosed with Alzheimer's, as high blood pressure causes damage to blood vessels in the brain. [19]

✓ **Depression:** Although researchers are working to clarify the mechanism of this relationship, depression is known to be a potential risk factor for provoking Alzheimer's.

✓ **Obesity:** Obesity increases the risk of developing type 2 diabetes, hypertension, and coronary events, making it a risk factor.

✓ **Hyperlipidemia:** This condition increases the risk of heart disease and cerebrovascular accidents, making it a risk factor for Alzheimer's.

✓ **Diet:** Diets high in carbohydrates and fats are seen as risk factors because they increase the risk of developing type 2 diabetes, hyperlipidemia, and coronary diseases.

✓ **Smoking:** Smoking is a risk factor for Alzheimer's because of the decrease in oxygen supply to the arteries that it causes.

✓ **Alcoholism:** Alcohol is neurotoxic, making it another risk factor for this disease.

✓ **Sedentary Lifestyle:** Lack of exercise may increase the likelihood of developing obesity and coronary diseases. Exercise stimulates the production of hormones that can improve memory and learning ability.

✓ **Stress:** Prolonged stress leads to high levels of cortisol production, which can cause brain damage by killing neurons and further provoking dementia.

✓ Social Isolation

✓ Hormonal Imbalance

✓ Vitamin Deficiency

X. PREVENTION

Prevention is defined as the measures used to prevent or delay the onset of a disease. In Alzheimer's disease, prevention plays a critical role, as indicated by research findings.[20] This chapter aims to educate and provide tools to reduce modifiable risks through prevention.

- ✓ **Active Lifestyle:** Research suggests that regular physical activity reduces the risk of developing Alzheimer's disease.[21] Physical activity offers numerous benefits, such as increasing lifespan, preventing premature deaths, and reducing the risk of coronary diseases, diabetes, and colorectal cancer.

- ✓ **Limit Alcohol Consumption:** Excessive alcohol consumption and alcoholism can lead to alterations in the brain and neuron death, potentially causing dementia.

- ✓ **STOP Smoking:** Smoking has been identified as a risk factor for developing dementia, as it increases the risk of coronary events and cerebrovascular accidents. While the exact reasons for this relationship are unclear, important physiological changes like decreased oxygen flow and increased oxidative stress contribute to neuronal damage. Smoking cessation improves circulation and oxygenation in the brain, reduces oxidative stress, and lowers the risk of dementia.

- ✓ **Control Your Blood Pressure:** Maintaining healthy blood pressure levels is crucial, as there is a link between high blood pressure and the development of Alzheimer's and other dementias.[19] Uncontrolled high blood pressure is a leading cause of vascular dementia, but it can be managed with medical treatment.[22]

- ✓ **Treat Your Depression:** Depression is the most common mental illness in both the United States and worldwide. It is a mental condition characterized by feelings of sadness, frequent crying, and a loss of interest in life. This is why patients diagnosed with this illness are at a higher risk of committing suicide. Depression is a condition that can often be improved or resolved through medical treatments. The most crucial aspect of dealing with this condition is identifying its symptoms and seeking professional help promptly. It's important to note that depression also increases a person's risk of developing dementia.

✓ **Control your Type II DM:** Research shows that elevated blood glucose levels predispose individuals to Alzheimer's. These changes in brain chemistry can lead to brain cell damage.

✓ **Maintain a Healthy Weight:** Maintaining a healthy weight is crucial because obesity increases the risk of developing both diabetes (DM) and coronary diseases. Being overweight or obese also raises the probability of developing Alzheimer's and other dementias.

✓ **Control Your Cholesterol:** High levels of cholesterol and triglycerides in the blood can raise the risk of dementia by interfering with the proper functioning of brain cells.

✓ **Decrease Stress:** Stress is a sensation of tension and anxiety that can arise from various situations or thoughts. Stress can have positive effects in small amounts, but when it starts to impact your daily life significantly, it becomes a medical condition that requires evaluation by a healthcare professional.

> ➤ The brain is the organ most affected by stress, as individuals experiencing stress tend to produce the hormone cortisol in higher quantities. Elevated cortisol levels can disrupt sleep patterns, lead to inflammation imbalances, affect blood sugar levels, and impair memory and concentration. Prolonged exposure to chronic stress is a known risk factor for developing Alzheimer's disease, underscoring the importance of managing stress levels.

✓ **Keep Healthy Sleep Habits:** Studies have shown that a lack of quality sleep is associated with an increased risk of dementia.[20] During sleep, the brain cleanses itself of toxic products. If we do not get adequate sleep, this natural process of eliminating these toxic products is hindered. As a result, there is an increased accumulation of Tau proteins and beta-amyloids, which are known to contribute to the development of Alzheimer's disease.[23] This underscores the importance of ensuring restful sleep.

✓ **Control Your Anxiety:** Anxiety is a state characterized by excessive bouts of worry that disrupt daily activities, hinder concentration, and lead to a continuous cycle of worrying. Studies have shown that there is a correlation between high anxiety levels and an increased risk of developing dementia.[24]

✓ **Eat Healthy:** Eating healthy is crucial for preventing Alzheimer's and other types of dementia. A balanced diet supports overall brain health by providing essential nutrients, reducing inflammation, and promoting cardiovascular health. Research suggests that diets rich in fruits, vegetables, whole grains, and lean proteins can help lower the risk of cognitive decline and Alzheimer's disease. Conversely, diets high in saturated fats, cholesterol, and processed foods may increase the risk. By adopting a healthy eating pattern, individuals can potentially safeguard themselves against the onset and progression of these debilitating conditions.

> ➢**DASH:** Focuses on fruits, vegetables, whole grains, lean proteins, and low-fat dairy products while limiting saturated fats, cholesterol, and sodium. It aims to reduce high blood pressure and promote heart health, potentially benefiting Alzheimer's patients by supporting brain health and reducing cardiovascular risk factors associated with cognitive decline.[21]

➢**Mediterranean Diet:** Rich in fruits, vegetables, whole grains, fish, olive oil, nuts, and seeds, with moderate consumption of poultry, dairy, and red wine. Associated with reduced risk of heart disease, stroke, and cognitive decline, its emphasis on healthy fats, antioxidants, and antiinflammatory compounds may help protect against Alzheimer's disease and other dementias by reducing oxidative stress, inflammation, and promoting cardiovascular health.[21]

✓ **Socialize:** Avoid social isolation, where individuals stop interacting with people outside their family environment. Recent studies have shown that isolation increases the risk of developing dementia.[25]

✓ Consult with your medical team about using vitamins, antioxidants, hormones, and foods such as strawberries, turmeric, ashwagandha, vitamin D, and COQ, among others.

✓ Avoid low oxygen levels at night.

✓ Avoid exposure to heavy metals like lead, cadmium, and mercury.

XI: STATISTICS <u>(AS OF 2023)</u>

1. *Over 6 million Americans live with Alzheimer's.*[17]

2. *In 2023, Alzheimer's & other dementias cost the nation an estimated 345 billion dollars.*[17]

3. *Alzheimer's is the 6th cause of death in the U.S.*[26]

4. *From 2000 to 2020, Alzheimer's-related deaths have increased to 145%. (Deaths related to cancer and cardiac diseases have decreased from 7 to 9%.).*[27]

5. *It is calculated that caregivers provide around 18.5 billion hours of care, valued at approximately $244 billion.*[28]

6. *Hispanics are 1.5x more predisposed to developing Alzheimer's than White Americans.*[29]

7. *Only four out of ten patients will speak with their doctors about their memory loss.*[17]

8. *82% of primary care physicians are the first line of defense for patients with Alzheimer's and other dementias.*[30]

9. *Women are more likely to develop Alzheimer's, comprising almost two-thirds of diagnosed cases among Americans.*[17]

10. *1 in 9 adults over the age of 65 have Alzheimer's.*[17]

11. *Alzheimer's is the 5th cause of death in patients over the age of 65.*[26]

12. *The estimated cost of the disease is projected to exceed $1.1 trillion by 2050.*[31]

13. *Over 11 million Americans provide unpaid care to people with Alzheimer's or other dementias.*[17]

14. *By 2050, it is estimated that more than 13 million individuals will live with Alzheimer's.*[17]

XII: FACTS (AS OF 2023)

1. Alzheimer's is the most common cause of dementia. (60%-70%).[5]

2. Alzheimer's is the 7th cause of death in the world.[5]

3. 1 in 3 elderly die of Alzheimer's and other dementias. (More patients die of Alzheimer's than of breast cancer and prostate cancer combined.) [17]

4. Every 65 seconds, someone is diagnosed with Alzheimer's in the U.S. [32]

5. Only 16% of elderly patients receive mental evaluations during primary care physician visits.[33]

6. Patients with Alzheimer's and other dementias carry double the risk of prolonged hospital stays.[17]

7. Elderly Black Americans carry 2x the likelihood of developing Alzheimer's when compared to elderly White Americans.[17]

8. A research study conducted in 2017 found that more than 60% of people with dementia were undiagnosed.[34]

9. Signs and symptoms of this disease may vary from person to person.[17]

10. Dementia is not a consequence of aging.

11. Dementia is one of the leading causes of disability and dependency in the U.S.[5]

12. *Finland is the country with the highest number of Alzheimer's patients.*[35]

13. *The disease typically lasts from 4 to 8 years but can last up to 20 years.*[36]

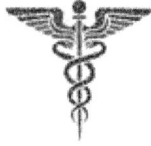

CHAPTER TWO

Stages of Alzheimer's: Symptoms, Complications & Recommendations

I. INTRODUCTION

ALZHEIMER'S DISEASE generally progresses slowly, affecting each patient differently. The duration of this illness varies from person to person, lasting approximately anywhere from 4 to 20 years.[36] Similarly, symptoms vary widely among individuals.

The variation in the duration of this illness and the diversity of symptom presentation depends on each diagnosed patient. Several models categorize the stages of Alzheimer's: the **7-stage model, 4-stage model** and **3-stage model**, among others. This variability results from the diverse clinical presentation of the disease.

Educating ourselves using these models, will help us respond appropriaely to changes and improve both the patients' and caregivers' quality of life. For the purpose of this guide, we will use the 3-stage model as our model of reference.

i. 3 Stage Model

✓ **Stage 1:** Mild (Early)
✓ **Stage 2:** Moderate (Middle)
✓ **Stage 3:** Severe (Late)

II. MILD OR EARLY STAGE

At this stage, individuals with Alzheimer's disease remain independent. The cognitive changes they experience do not hinder their daily activities, including bathing, eating, or their ability to work.[36]

i. **Symptoms:** The initial symptoms of this disease present during this stage. In most cases, the patient can maintain their independence, requiring minimal assistance from their caregiver.

> ✓ Recent memory loss accompanied by repetitive statements or questions.

> ✓ Problems with cognitive abilities, such as impaired judgment and decision-making.

> ✓ Misplacement of valuable objects.

> ✓ Difficulty recalling the names of familiar individuals outside of immediate family.

> ✓ Easily becoming disoriented, especially while driving

> ✓ Language and communication difficulties, including trouble recalling specific words.

> ✓ Potential signs of depression.

> ✓ Disturbances in sleep patterns.

> ✓ Accidental skipping of meals despite maintaining a generally healthy appetite.

> ✓ Behavioral changes such as irritability, agitation, or aggression.

> ✓ Personality shifts, potentially exhibiting antisocial behavior or the use of inappropriate language.

> ✓ Difficulty planning and solving mathematical problems.

ii. Complications

✓ Forgetting medical appointments which can disrupt their healthcare routine and lead to missed treatments or screenings.

✓ Repeatedly asking the location of items such as car keys, indicating shortterm memory loss.

✓ Neglecting financial responsibilities, potentially resulting in monetary difficulties or unpaid bills.

✓ Making withdrawals from savings accounts without recollection, hinting at impaired financial judgment.

✓ Experiencing strained relationships with neighbors and friends due to behavioral changes or forgetfulness.

✓ Forgetting to take prescribed medications, compromising their health management, and exacerbating medical conditions.

✓ Becoming disoriented or lost while driving, posing safety risks to themselves and others.

✓ Failing to remember important events, contributing to feelings of sadness or depression.

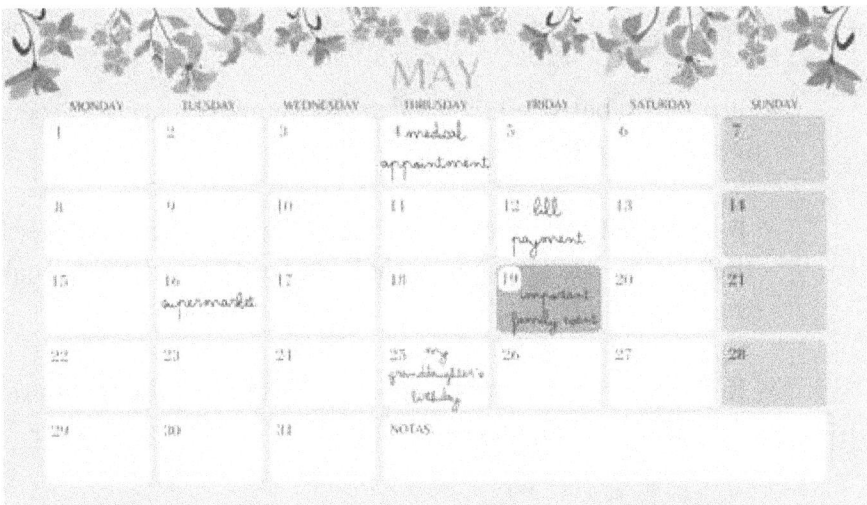

iii. Recommendations

✓ Do not ignore symptoms (they may not be part of the normal aging process).

✓ Seek immediate help from a healthcare professional.

✓ Show empathy, listen actively, and be patient, treating others as you would like to be treated.

✓ Keep monthly or weekly planners accessible to the patient.

✓ Keep calendars visible and record medical appointments, family events, birthdays, payday dates, and other important dates.

✓ Organize and label things so the patient does not have to ask about them constantly.

✓ Discuss legal matters, financials, power of attorneys, advanced directives, and wills, among other things. This can help to avoid discourse between family members. Failing to do so could create problems when making decisions for the patient.

✓ Help to establish exercise routines.

✓ Promote a balanced diet and assist them in creating a grocery list, weekly menus, and a recipe book.

✓ Respect patients' preferences: If patients prefer to shower in the evening, do not change their preferences, as it may make them resistant.

✓ Reduce patients' resistance to care by treating them with respect, love, and dignity.

✓ Encourage independence and guide them in activities, avoiding phrases like *"YOU CAN'T."*

✓ Provide information instead of asking lengthy questions, as excessive questions can overwhelm the patient.

✓ Avoid embarrassing the patient or making a scene of their forgetfulness or mistakes.

✓ Do not contradict the patient; find an alternative to achieve the desired result.

✓ Establish Routines, which can help reduce the patient's anxiety and depression by giving them a sense of predictability. [37]

✓ Consider implementing a meal routine to ensure they remember to eat.

✓ All routines must be flexible to avoid causing stress and tailored to the patient's preferences.

✓ If the patient encounters someone they haven't seen in a while, take the initiative to mention the person's name first. For example, you can say, *"Hi Isabel, how are you?"* This can help the patient remember the person's name.

✓ A simple smile can convey love and warmth, reducing the patient's frustration.

✓ Treat the patient patiently and consider how you would like to be treated.

✓ When engaging in activities with the patient, try to move at a slower pace to accommodate their needs.

✓ Financial supervision: Monitor the patient's bank accounts and routine payments to manage their responsibilities effectively.

✓ Take charge of coordinating, supervising, and following up on medical appointments and treatments. Consider using a pillbox to organize medications.

✓ If the patient forgets a word while speaking, help them remember without causing embarrassment.

✓ Obtain a labeled pillbox that indicates the day and frequency of medications.

✓ When necessary, lessen the patient's responsibilities. For instance, if they are going on vacation, thoroughly review all of the necessary details to ensure they remember everything.

✓ Avoid embarrassing the patient in front of others or making a spectacle of their forgetfulness.

✓ Take on the supervision of tasks the patient managed, such as car inspections, insurance renewals, and mail handling.

III. MODERATE STAGE:

The moderate stage is typically the longest phase, during which the patient requires increased supervision to carry out their daily activities. They become more dependent on the caretaker and can no longer live independently.[36] It's important to note that symptoms can vary from patient to patient. The next step is to identify any signs that might lead to complications.

i. *Symptoms*

✓ Individuals become increasingly forgetful, often repeating themselves.

✓ The patient is unable to may experience speech problems, leading to difficulty in communication.

✓ The patient cannot operate a vehicle safely.

✓ Incontinence problems.

✓ Personality changes, such as irritability, become noticeable.

✓ Patients may stop participating in hobbies and social activities they once enjoyed.

✓ Increased dependency on others for daily tasks.

✓ Refusal to complete essential responsibilities such as showering.

✓ The patient forgets their medical appointments, family events, and birthdays.

✓ They may forget to follow through with their prescribed medical treatments.

✓ Physical changes, like muscle weakness, may lead to weight loss and reduced appetite, making them more prone to falls.

✓ Psychiatric symptoms: Such as hallucinations, aggression, delirium, depression, agitation, and delusions, among other symptoms.

✓ Patients may struggle when using silverware, resorting to eating with their hands.

✓ Perception problems: for example, the patient cannot interpret road signs, making driving dangerous.

✓ Sleep disturbances.

✓ The patient may begin to experience difficulty recognizing close family members.

✓ Disorientation in person, time, and space at a frequent rate.

✓ Behavioral changes, they may begin to behave in a socially unacceptable way.

✓ Repetitive actions, such as walking from one side to another or hitting a spot repetitively.

✓ Difficulty completing tasks.

✓ Inappropriate sexual behaviors: the patient may confuse a stranger with their partner.

✓ The patient stops speaking but does so in a way that hides their symptoms.

✓ Difficulty differentiating between sarcasm and social cues.

ii. Complications

✓ Patients are more susceptible to falls at this stage.

✓ Weight loss may occur.

✓ Longer hospital stays may occur as a result of deteriorating medical conditions caused by the patient forgetting to follow their medical treatment.

✓ Patients may misuse their medications, potentially causing medication overdoses.

✓ They may try to attack the caregiver because of psychiatric manifestations that make them believe they're getting attacked.

✓ The patient is at a higher risk of developing mental illnesses such as depression, anxiety, hallucinations, etc.

✓ They may be more susceptible to bedsores due to spending long periods seated or resting in the same exact position.

✓ Difficulty using silverware can lead to decreased food intake.

✓ Patients are easily distracted and have a hard time paying attention.

✓ The caregiver may become exhausted as the patient acts like a shadow, following them around.

✓ Increase wandering behavior.

✓ They may try to *"elope."*

✓ The patient may become frustrated when they cannot communicate what they're trying to say. They may become aggressive, anxious, etc., as a form of alternate communication.

✓ Increased likelihood of dehydration, UTIs, and pneumonia.

✓ They become irritable if they go to a social activity where they do not recognize many people.

✓ The patient is more likely to choke and develop pneumonia as a result of aspiration.

✓ The patient may attack their caregiver or loved ones.

✓ The patient may need to be taken to a mental institution because of manifesting psychiatric illnesses.

✓ They may cause the death of a bystander if they continue to drive a vehicle.

✓ The patient is ashamed of their forgetfulness and refuses to interact with others.

iii. Recommendations

✓ Use tablecloths of a single color without designs. The patient has difficulty seeing and understanding reality, so they may confuse the designs on the tablecloth with edible items. Avoid plates with designs for the same reason.

✓ Offer the patient foods they can eat with their hands to erase the stress of using flatware.

✓ Lighting is vital during this stage, as the patient may wander at night. Having visibly lit rooms can help prevent falls.

✓ Avoid messy hallways, as this can also cause accidents.

✓ Avoid exposing patients to situations where they no longer act according to social standards. These situations may leave the patient frustrated.

✓Organization is essential so that the patient can function for a longer period.

✓Label as many things as possible; this helps the patient feel more productive and decreases frustration.

✓Respect the patient's preferences; for example, if the patient does not like showering during the evening, then help them maintain that routine and help them shower in the morning.

✓During this stage, judgment is severely affected, and the patient should not be left alone in the kitchen as they may touch the hot stove or other dangerous items.

✓Maintain all firearms or dangerous objects away from the reach of the patient, as they could use those items against their caregivers or other loved ones. Psychiatric hallucinations being one of the possible dangerous triggers.

✓Hire someone to handle their daily needs, such as preparing food, showering, and other house tasks.

✓Avoid all distractions during dinner time. This includes television and other loud, distracting noises.

✓To help avoid any incontinence accidents, make sure to label the bathroom.

✓Create a bathroom routine every 2–3 hours and do not wait for the patient to tell you they need to use the restroom.

✓Avoid big gatherings and keep events family-only.

✓Consult with their doctor in the case of any psychiatric complications.

✓Offer them water every 2 hours to avoid dehydration.

✓Continually keep track of their bowel movements.

✓Identify yourself with the patient whenever you approach them in any way.

✓Explain each task to the patient beforehand so that they know what is happening. This helps avoid any agitation of frustration in the patient.

✓Smile!

✓Be patient and tolerant.

✓Refrain from doing tasks for them in a rushed and rough way.

✓Place an identifying accessory on them, such as a bracelet, chip, or any other type of tracking device engraved with information, in case the patient gets lost.

✓Avoid infantilizing the patient and treating them like a child.

✓Ensure the house is closed at all times and keep the key hidden to prevent the patient from wandering and getting lost.

✓Paint rooms in bright colors.

✓Keep rooms clean and organized.

IV. LATE OR SEVERE STAGE

During the severe stage, the patient loses independence and cannot perform the most basic daily tasks. They cannot live alone anymore, and their survival entirely relies on their caregiver.[36] This stage poses significant challenges for family members as the patient no longer recognizes them, demanding great effort and dedication from the caregivers. To navigate this stage effectively, caregivers should focus on minimizing complications by educating themselves and providing exceptional care.

As cognitive deterioration progresses, this stage ultimately leads to the final stage, where the patient approaches the end of their life. The following chapter will delve into the final stage in depth.

i. *Symptoms*

✓ Difficulty remembering their caregiver or family members.

✓ They are unable to communicate effectively and only say words and phrases, not complete sentences. To express themselves, they may use other methods of communication, such as screaming, cursing, scratching, biting, kicking, etc.

✓ Muscle weakness that makes walking and sitting difficult; mainly, they are either in a wheelchair or bedridden.

✓ Problems swallowing and choking.

✓ Weight and muscle loss due to diet changes.

✓ The patient most likely spends long periods sleeping and is more susceptible to bedsores.

✓ The patient depends entirely on the caregiver, who must complete 100% of the patient's daily needs. These include showering, eating, etc.

✓ Fecal and urinary incontinence.

✓ As a result of cognitive damage, patients suffer psychiat-ric conditions such as hallucinations, psychosis, delirium, aggression, and anxiety, among others.

✓ The patient is more susceptible to falls and suffers mainly from hip fractures, which are caused when caregivers try to move or transfer the patient.

✓ The patient depends on diapers as a means to address urinary incontinence.

✓ Dry skin and capillary fragility

✓ Fungal infections or dermatitis in the genital area, underarms, neck, fingers, and toes.

ii. *Complications*

✓ Higher susceptibility to urinary infections as a result of urinary incontinence and low fluid intake.

✓ Higher likelihood of developing bedsores due to long periods sitting in a wheelchair or bedridden, coupled with urinary incontinence.

✓ Increased pain levels caused by ulcers and muscle weakness, among other symptoms.

✓ The patient displays ankyloses (Stiffness of a joint), making diaper changes and personal hygiene more difficult.

✓ Increased susceptibility to pneumonia caused by aspiration, which results from problems swallowing and choking due to muscle weakness.

✓ As a consequence of tone and muscle loss, the patient cannot hold their neck up.

✓ Diaper use may cause ulcers and infections if they are not changed frequently.

✓ Chronic medical conditions could potentially worsen due to the patient experiencing difficulty swallowing their medications.

✓ Hospitalizations are more frequent thanks to caregivers' difficulty in identifying signs and symptoms of medical complications.

✓ Skin becomes dry and creates bruises due to skin dryness and capillary fragility.

✓ The caregiver can become infected with dermatitis, colds or others health conditions if they do not protect themselves with gloves or masks.

✓ Weight loss continues to increase.

✓ Difficulty tolerating regular food consistencies, which may lead to choking.

✓ Dental hygiene is poor due to the patient's difficulty visiting the dentist.

✓ They are at a high risk of falling if the bed rails are left down.

iii. Recommendations

✓ Evaluate signs of dysphagia, where the patient cannot swallow, and notify their health provider for treatment if necessary.

✓ During this stage, hygiene is essential to avoid ulcers and secondary dermatitis. Therefore, disposable diapers should be checked every 2 hours and changed when needed.

✓ When changing diapers, use barriers protective creams to help prevent ulcers.

✓ The caregiver must stay alert to notify the health provider if the patient has stopped eating, has a fever, or any other manifestations of pain in order to seek immediate care.

✓ Patients should use items that help their care and management, such as a hospital bed and wheelchair.

✓ Bed rails should stay up at all times to help prevent falls.

✓ The caregiver should coordinate a medical at-home visit because the patient most likely cannot attend medical appointments.

✓ The caregiver is responsible for providing the patient with their medications.

✓ Apply creams to the dry skin to help avoid complications. Constantly evaluate the state of their skin.

✓ Follow bowel and urine movements to avoid intestinal obstructions as a result of constipation or urinary infections.

✓ Use pillows between their legs and other protective materials to help prevent bedsores and contact with bony prominences such as the knees, heels, elbows, etc. Some examples include the use of air mattresses or gel pillows.

✓ When bathing the patient, dry them well to avoid fungal infections in the genital area, underarms, neck, fingers, and toes.

✓ In order to help protect dry skin with capillary fragility, try to avoid creams and soaps that have fragrances or alcohol in them.

✓ When applying creams, if the skin is intact, give them gentle massages to stimulate circulation and make the patient feel loved.

✓ Wheelchair patients should be repositioned every 2 hours.

✓ Provide a diet that follows the instructions of their healthcare provider.

✓ The caregiver must protect both patients and their own health by using gloves when changing diapers, bathing them, or managing secretions.

✓ Whenever you intervene with a patient, wash your hands before and after every interaction.

✓ Consult with your healthcare provider to see if the patient needs a different food consistency due to the patient's dysphagia.

✓ Always verify food temperatures before feeding the patient.

✓ Verify with your healthcare professional if nutritional supplements would benefit the patient.

✓ Verify with your health care professional, if food thickener would help their diet and prevent aspiration pneumonias.

✓ During this and all stages, respect the preferences of the patient with Alzheimer's or other dementias.

✓ Avoid leaving the patient alone while changing their diaper or bathing them; the rails should always stay up to help prevent falls.

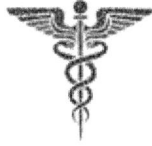

CHAPTER THREE

Final Stage

I. INTRODUCTION

ALZHEIMER'S IS AN ILLNESS that has no cure. During the severe stage, the patient enters the final stage as cognitive deterioration worsens. In this final stage, the patient will present certain signs and symptoms that will indicate that the last days are near. Treatment will focus on decreasing pain and creating a comfortable environment for the patient.

In this chapter, we'll go over the importance of planning the patient's future. Advanced directives and power of attorney are important documents that we should have ready with our lawyers to avoid uncomfortable situations.

During this final stage, the caregiver and the rest of the family will experience the suffering of seeing how the light in your loved one's life is dimming. It is important to find spiritual and psychological help from your healthcare team to help guide you through the final stage of your loved one.

II. SIGNS & SYMPTOMS THE END IS NEAR

In patients with Alzheimer's or other dementias, the signs and symptoms that the end is near vary from patient to patient, as does the duration of the stage.

i. *Most Common Signs*

- ✓ Difficulty when swallowing or chewing.
- ✓ Long periods asleep
- ✓ Unresponsive
- ✓ Cold and cyanotic extremities
- ✓ Labored breathing
- ✓ Grey-toned skin
- ✓ Difficulty verbalizing
- ✓ Difficulty urinating as a result of kidney failure.
- ✓ Immobile
- ✓ 24/7 care and attention to their needs
- ✓ Multiple infections, with the potential for antibiotic resistance.
- ✓ Increased pain levels
- ✓ Altered vital signs, including pulse rate, temperature, blood pressure, oxygen saturation, and heart rate.
- ✓ Hallucinations
- ✓ Unconsciousness
- ✓ Altered mental state
- ✓ Cheyne-Stokes Respiration, which is an irregular pattern of breathing.

III. END OF LIFE CARE

During this final stage, care is focused on minimizing pain and making the patient's last days as comfortable as possible. It is important to understand that the patient is not hungry or thirsty because the body is preparing itself for the end.

i. Recommendations for Care

- ✓ Focus on minimizing pain.
- ✓ Family members need to respect the patient's advanced directives and medical decisions.
- ✓ Maintain their environment as comfortable as possible.
- ✓ Understand that the patient is not hungry and does not feel any pain.
- ✓ Play soft and calming music in their room.
- ✓ Keep lights dim.
- ✓ Give them hand and foot massages.
- ✓ If the patient cannot swallow, do not keep insisting and pressuring them.
- ✓ Artificial feeding is not recommended because the potential for complications such as pressure ulcers and aspiration pneumonia.[38]
- ✓ Always use gloves when changing diapers or bathing the patient.
- ✓ It is important to be present, talk to them, say everything is okay, and reassure them you and the rest of their family will be okay.
- ✓ It is crucial to forgive anything that needs to be forgiven.
- ✓ Pay attention to signs of pain such as facial expressions, eyebrow movements, complaints, or cries. When you observe these signs, give them the pain medications provided by their healthcare.
- ✓ Notify family members that the patient is in the finally stage, so that they may say goodbye. If a family member wishes to refrain from saying their goodbyes, allow them to make that decision.

✓ Take care of their personal and oral hygiene and change diapers every 2 hours. Maintain their lips moist all the time.
✓ Verify that the room temperature is appropriate and comfortable.
✓ Respect the patient's wishes. Always making sure to respect their religious preferences and avoid being biased by your own opinion.
✓ Only the closest relatives should be in the room at the final moment. This helps ensure the patient remains comfortable during the end.

At a certain point during this final stage, patients may exhibit brief periods of lucidity. While it is important to take advantage of these moments, it is crucial to understand that they are temporary and are not a sign that the patient's health is improving.[39] Instead, these moments offer an opportunity for meaningful connection and communication with the patient, allowing caregivers to enjoy the clarity that the patient may briefly exhibit. By recognizing and valuing these moments, caregivers can provide comfort and support to both the patient and their loved ones, fostering a sense of peace and dignity in the final stages of their journey.

IV. ADVANCED DIRECTIVES

Advanced directives are medical decisions stipulated in a legal document by a person of old age who maintains legal capacity. In this document, the individual states the care they would like to receive in the case of physical or mental incapacity, and whether they would like to receive medical treatment.

This document should be shared among the family, legal guardian, and medical team so that their medical decisions may be respected. The importance of the advanced directives is that their wishes will be respected in the case of incapacity, and family members will not have to be responsible for making difficult decisions. This document also stipulates other wishes, such as organ donation, autopsies, and cremation. This document will help avoid the need for court intervention.

i. Treatment Options

> - Hospice
> - Artificial feeding
> - Palliative care
> - Resuscitation or DNAR (Do Not Attempt Resuscitation)
> - Hospitalization

V. MEDICAL DECISIONS

Here, we will discuss medical decisions regarding treating a patient with Alzheimer's or other dementias during their final days. During the final stage, the patient presents signs and symptoms that help predict the end. During this time, their healthcare team will explain the different medical treatment options available so that you may make your medical decision. In an ideal world, the patient would already have advanced directives, but unfortunately, that is not always the case.

i. Most Common Medical Decisions

✓ **Hospice:** This type of healthcare facility is typically ordered by a medical provider in cases where patients are in a terminal stage for a condition with no cure. The patient's life expectancy must be less than six months.[40] The aim is for treatment to minimize pain and offer comfortable care for the patient at home with no need for a hospital.

✓ **Palliative Care:** This is a type of healthcare geared towards patients who have received a diagnosis of a grave illness and are currently receiving treatment through which they can be cured. The aim of this type of care is to improve the patient's quality of life.[40] This type of care can be provided in hospitals, at home, or nursing homes.

➢ **Hospice vs. Palliative Care:** In hospice, the patient has a disease with no cure and a life expectancy of less than six months. In palliative care, the patient can be cured and recover fully. [40]

✓ **Artificial Feeding:** When the patient with Alzheimer's or other dementias is at the final stage, they cannot eat or swallow due to muscle weakness. At this time, the medical provider will offer the option of artificial feeding. Artificial feeding is administered via a nasogastric tube (NGT) or a Percutaneous endoscopic gastrostomy tube (PEG) placed in the stomach.[41]

> ➤ **Medical Opinion:** From a medical perspective, artificial feeding is not recommended. Studies show that it may even decrease patient survival. This option may cause pressure ulcers and increase the risk of aspiration pneumonia.[38] If the patient has a history of agitation, the medical provider will order a physical restraint for their extremities to limit their movements and prevent them from disrupting the tube.

✓ **<u>Cardiopulmonary Resuscitation (CPR):</u>** Patients who are in a terminal stage and need to be admitted to the hospital will be asked if they want to be resuscitated or not in the case of an emergency. Resuscitation, or "CPR" is a technique to bring patients back to life when their heart or respiration has stopped. If the patient has advanced directives, the wishes listed on the document will be followed. Otherwise, the family members or legal guardian will be responsible for making the decision.

✓ **<u>Hospitalization:</u>** In the case of a patient with recurrent infections, it is possible for the healthcare team to explain that the patient has stopped responding to antibiotics due to a developed resistance to them. In this case, relatives or the legal guardian may decide whether they want the patient hospitalized.

Educating ourselves on the final stage of the illness can help us make decisions that benefit the diagnosed patient. Surrounding ourselves with an empathetic healthcare team and being informed of each stage of the disease is the best recommendation for our loved ones.

VI. ACCEPTANCE AND GRIEF

i. Acceptance

Accepting that death is a natural and inevitable process is vital for both the caregiver and the relatives of the loved one. Accepting death does not mean that you're minimizing the suffering of the loss of your loved one. Being educated helps decrease anxiety and fear of the unknown, which helps us make decisions that benefit that individual.

For patients with Alzheimer's, the most important thing for their final days is to make them as pain-free and comfortable as possible. They should be surrounded only by people who love them and shower them with love and affection. Accepting that death is inevitable helps us say goodbye and let them go. Sometimes, it even almost permits them, in a way, to leave, knowing that the people they are leaving behind will be okay and grateful for the love that they gave.

ii. Grief

Grief is the emotional process that we confront when we lose a loved one. Each person experiences it and responds differently. Grief can be expressed in many ways, mainly physically and emotionally, while also having different stages. The important key to surviving grief is to seek help from a spiritual counselor, relatives, and your healthcare team to face the grief head-on and prevent it from developing into a mental illness. Therefore, staying educated and seeking help when needed is essential.

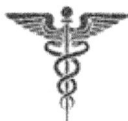

CHAPTER FOUR

Being a Caregiver

I. INTRODUCTION

BEING A CAREGIVER many times is not a choice; sometimes circumstances force us to accept the responsibility of being a caregiver. A lack of information and understanding about Alzheimer's provokes anxiety, confusion, and disorientation.

The latest statistics from the U.S. Department of Health report that 83% of caregivers for Alzheimer's patients are family members; most of these caregivers lack the proper training to take care of a patient, which complicates their care.

It's important to decrease frustration and disorientation by educating ourselves, and thus avoiding the physical and mental wear and tear that caregivers experience. In the following pages, we'll review some concepts of being a good caregiver and more important tools to help avoid caregiver burnout. In this way, we can help offer the best care possible for the patient.

II. ARE YOU A CAREGIVER?

Being a caregiver entails many responsibilities, from purchasing groceries to coordinating medical appointments and assisting with daily activities. It's a role that requires dedication and compassion. As we immerse ourselves in this caregiving journey, we must acknowledge our challenges and the importance of self-education about the condition affecting our loved one.

Caring for someone with a diagnosed condition, especially one requiring round-the-clock supervision, is no small task. It demands not only physical effort but also emotional resilience. Understanding the intricacies of the disease not only enhances our ability to provide quality care but also equips us to identify the signs of caregiver burnout—a state that can profoundly affect both the caregiver and the patient.

Amid this demanding role, it's vital to recognize our limits and prioritize our well-being. It's perfectly acceptable to reassess our capabilities and acknowledge when we need additional support. As the disease progresses and the demands of caregiving increase, it's okay to admit when we can no longer provide the level of care our loved one requires.

Saying *"I CAN'T"* doesn't diminish our dedication or love for the patient, but underscores our commitment to their best interests. Deciding to seek alternative care options or consider placement in a healthcare facility is challenging. Still, ultimately, it may be the most compassionate choice for both the patient and the caregiver. In prioritizing our well-being, we ensure we can continue to provide the best possible care for our loved ones, even if it means seeking help from others or transitioning to a different caregiving arrangement.

III. DECIDING TO BE A CAREGIVER

Often, the decision to step into the role of a caregiver is not simply a matter of choice but a response to circumstances that compel individuals to care for their loved ones. Whether it's a parent, spouse, friend, or another cherished individual, social expectations, norms, and a deep sense of love or duty can drive one to take on the responsibility of caregiving. Whatever the underlying reasons, we need to be honest with ourselves about our commitment. If we embrace this role, we must fully assume its responsibilities. This means equipping ourselves with knowledge and preparing diligently to offer the highest standard of care to those suffering from Alzheimer's disease or other forms of dementia.

Initially, the caregiver is driven by a genuine desire, love, and willingness to care for a loved one diagnosed with Alzheimer's or dementia. However, as the disease progresses and cognitive abilities decline, the patient's dependence on the caregiver often intensifies. This shift can lead to what is known as caregiver burnout, which can take a toll on both the caregiver's physical and mental well-being. It is imperative to recognize the signs of burnout, a topic we will delve into further in the subsequent pages of this book. Acknowledging one's limitations and considering alternative care options are crucial steps toward ensuring the overall well-being of the caregiver and the patient.

As we navigate the complexities of caregiving, it's essential to understand that it's not just a single decision but rather an ongoing journey filled with challenges and rewards. By arming ourselves with knowledge, practicing self-awareness, and seeking support when needed, we can strive to provide compassionate and effective care to those entrusted to our care.

IV: TRAITS OF A GOOD CAREGIVER

As you embark on the journey of caregiving, it's essential to understand that you've chosen a role of immense importance and responsibility. As you fulfill the duties of a caregiver, it's crucial to recognize the inherent duality of your existence—you are not only a caregiver but also a human being with your own needs and desires.

While dedicating yourself to the care of others, it's easy to lose sight of your well-being. However, maintaining your physical and emotional health is paramount. Remember, by taking care of yourself, you are better equipped to provide exceptional care to those entrusted to your care, particularly patients with Alzheimer's or other forms of dementia.

Being a dedicated caregiver means being attuned to your own needs as well. Recognize the signs of fatigue and exhaustion and address them promptly. Prioritizing your self-care ensures you can consistently provide the high-quality care that your patients deserve.

In the demanding role of a caregiver, you must nurture yourself as much as you do others. Whether finding moments of respite, engaging in activities that bring you joy, or seeking support from friends and family, remember that your well-being directly impacts the quality of care you provide.

By acknowledging your humanity and prioritizing self-care, you safeguard your health and enhance your ability to support and care for individuals with dementia compassionately. Embrace this journey with a commitment to your patients and yourself, knowing you become an even more effective caregiver by nurturing yourself.

✓ Patience, flexibility, and Creativity

✓ Sense of Humor

✓ Positive Attitude

✓ Respectful

✓ Has a soft voice, smiles, and is friendly

✓ Avoids sarcasm

✓ Maintains eye contact.

✓ Asks brief questions.

✓ Constantly identify themselves to the patient.

✓ Completes tasks slowly.

✓ Desire to learn and educate themselves.

✓ Organization

✓ Maintains routines and is well organized

✓ Provides care with dignity, respect, and love.

✓ Provides a balanced diet.

✓ Encourages exercise and healthy movement.

✓ Relaxes and practices self-care.

✓ Respects the patient's decisions and preferences.

✓ Completes routine health checks for both themselves and the patient.

✓ Says, *"I CAN'T, or I NEED HELP,"* when they feel exhausted.

✓ Avoid infantilizing the patient and refer to them by their names instead of pet names or nicknames.

✓ Promote the patient's independence as much as possible. However, do not force the Alzheimer's patient to do tasks they are unable to complete.

V. RESPONSIBILITIES OF A GOOD CAREGIVER

Being responsible caregivers means offering quality and excellent care for the patient. The caregiver must follow through on their obligations and the patient's needs. Consequently, they are tasked with ensuring the physical and mental well-being of the patient.

In caregiving, the caregiver is the primary facilitator of the patient's care journey. They must execute their duties diligently and with compassion, ensuring that every aspect of the patient's care plan is meticulously carried out. This entails attending to the patient's immediate needs and proactively identifying and addressing any potential challenges or concerns that may arise.

Moreover, the caregiver's responsibility extends beyond the physical realm to encompass the emotional and psychological dimensions of care. Caregiver's provide comfort, support, reassurance, and companionship to the patient in times of distress or uncertainty. By fostering a nurturing and compassionate environment, caregivers play a pivotal role in promoting the well-being of those under their care.

- ✓ Provide a safe environment.
- ✓ Continuously monitor the patient's symptoms, including pain, stress, dehydration, and cognitive deterioration.
- ✓ Promptly notify the healthcare team of any changes to facilitate necessary treatment.
- ✓ Coordinate medical care for the patient.
- ✓ Respect the patient's medical decisions.
- ✓ Educate themselves about the disease.
- ✓ Take care of themselves physically and emotionally.
- ✓ Seek help when necessary.
- ✓ Offer an environment rich in cognitively stimulating activities.
- ✓ Promote exercise.
- ✓ Offer a balanced diet.

✓ Rest

✓ Keep up with their social lives and hobbies.

✓ Take care of their health and continue any medical treatments.

✓ Obtain helpful tools such as calendars, digital clocks, memory games, phones with large keyboards, walkers, hospital beds, etc.

✓ Coordinate with trained personnel to provide the patient with cognitive, multisensorial, and psychomotor therapies to decrease cognitive deterioration.

VI. SIGNS OF CAREGIVER BURNOUT

Being the primary caregiver for a loved one in need of round-the-clock care is a job that is an incredibly rewarding yet demanding responsibility. The tireless commitment and sacrifice of caregivers often lead to what is commonly termed *"caregiver burnout."* This phenomenon is characterized by overwhelming exhaustion, both physically and emotionally, resulting from the relentless demands of caregiving without adequate support or respite.

Recognizing the signs of caregiver burnout is crucial for the well-being of both the caregiver and the care recipient. Symptoms may manifest in various forms, such as persistent fatigue, feelings of isolation or loneliness, irritability, changes in appetite or sleep patterns, and neglecting one's health needs.

Caregivers must prioritize their own well-being and seek help when necessary. This might involve contacting family members or support groups, consulting healthcare professionals for guidance, or exploring respite care options to allow for much-needed rest and rejuvenation. By acknowledging the signs of caregiver burnout and taking proactive steps to address them, caregivers can ensure they continue to provide the best possible care while safeguarding their health and well-being.

i. *Signs of Caregiver Burnout*

- ✓ Frequent crying
- ✓ Low energy levels
- ✓ Sleep problems or difficulty getting out of bed
- ✓ Poor/Increased appetite
- ✓ Social isolation
- ✓ Depression-like symptoms
- ✓ Strong emotional experiences:
  - ➤ Frustration or irritability
  - ➤ Anxiety
  - ➤ Sadness, rage, crying episodes, etc.
  - ➤ Eating disorders
  - ➤ Low energy levels

VII. DEPRESSION: MOST COMMON COM-PLICATION

Depression is a psychiatric illness where the patient experiences sadness, irritability, guilt, insomnia, low energy levels, difficulty concentrating, tiredness, behavioral changes, headaches, and digestive issues, among other symptoms. However, the most concerning symptom of depression is suicidal ideation. According to the World Health Organization (WHO), approximately 5% of adults suffer from depression, which is the first cause of disability in the U.S.[42] The key problem is that a very high percentage of patients with depression do not seek help.

Caregivers for patients with Alzheimer's are susceptible to depression, as seen by the latest statistics. Caregivers can suffer from burnout, which is characterized by anxiety, overwhelming feelings of sadness, irritability, and apathy, among others.[43] As the disease progresses, the patient becomes more dependent on the caregiver, which can cause feelings of stress for the caregiver, which can eventually complicate feelings of depression. [44]

The main idea of this section is for you to identify the signs and symptoms of depression so that you may seek the professional help you require. In that way, you can ensure you are in the best state to provide patients with the quality of care they need.

VIII. RECOMMENDATIONS FOR A BURNED-OUT CAREGIVER

Taking care of a patient is difficult, but taking care of an Alzheimer's or dementia patient is even more complicated. The responsibility is much more demanding. Because of cognitive deterioration, memory loss, lack of judgment, poor reasoning, and other things, the patient becomes dependent on the caregiver. Providing care backed by knowledge of the disease is IMPORTANT for this type of patient.

To effectively care for a patient with Alzheimer's, the attitude we adopt is crucial for success as caregivers. It is important to recognize that the patient is experiencing a medical condition known as anosognosia. This condition renders the patient unaware and incapable of understanding the reality of their illness and mental state. As a result, they may refuse treatment and lack consciousness.

Caregivers should understand that patients do not do these things to upset them. Instead, it's essential to recognize that these individuals are unwell and experiencing cognitive deterioration due to improper brain functioning. This, in turn, leads to the behavioral changes they exhibit. This type of patient progressively deteriorates and is not oriented in time, place, or person, meaning they live in their own worlds.

In conclusion, individuals with Alzheimer's or other forms of dementia may display various behavioral changes, leading to a 24/7 dependency on caregivers and ultimately resulting in caregiver burnout. A significant number of caregivers for such patients often experience mental health issues, such as depression. One of the primary objectives of this guide is to prevent depression by providing guidance and the necessary tools to identify early stages, encouraging caregivers to seek help, and avoiding burnout.

i. Recommendations for Burned-Out Caregivers

✓ Ask for help from other family members so you can take time for yourself.

✓ Employ someone to assist you with patient care, allowing you to spend enough time on your hobbies, personal pursuits, and medical needs.

✓ Use relaxation techniques, including meditation, yoga, and exercise, for both you and the patient.

✓ Participating in a caregiver support group, whether online or in person, can be beneficial. Interacting with other caregivers and sharing experiences can help prevent feelings of isolation.[45]

✓ Relocate the patient to a long-term care home.

✓ Take the patient to daycare from 8 am–5 pm.

✓ Seek help from healthcare professionals: neurologists, primary care physicians, and psychiatrists.

✓ Stimulate cognitive, motor, physical, and cognitive areas to improve the patient's quality of life and help decrease caregiver burnout.

IX. THE DECISION

"Decision" refers to the choice between several options. In our personal experience, the decision to place our father in a long-term care home made us feel sad and frustrated. The lack of specialized care homes for patients with memory problems made the decision even more challenging. However, in hindsight, we understand we were wrong.

Initially, our mother became his caregiver, not by choice, and the circumstances of his diagnosis led to her being his caregiver for years. Unfortunately, his cognitive deterioration was progressing, and taking care of him at home became harder. As his children, we tried different alternatives to help in his care, but the distance and our personal lives made it difficult to help support him. We used all of our resources to hire personnel, but complications and his behavioral changes made it impossible for them, which always resulted in them quitting. Our mother was exhausted physically and mentally and was presenting with symptoms of caregiver burnout, and we, as her children, had to act fast. We analyzed all of the available options that would benefit them both, decided to place him in a long-term care home.

The decision to place him in a nursing home was and will always be one of the saddest and most difficult decisions of our lives. We understand that putting patients in these long-term nursing homes is a responsible decision. Today, as their children, we feel pleased with our decision, which helped prevent the physical and mental deterioration of our mother that she would have experienced due to caregiver burnout. It is our responsibility as caregivers or loved ones of a patient with Alzheimer's or other dementias to recognize when we feel symptoms of burnout and to evaluate the different care options available, always making the best decision for the benefit of both the patient and the caregiver.

X. FREE YOURSELF FROM THE GUILT

"Guilt" is a feeling that has a negative effect on our lives and causes us to feel ill. Traditionally, culturally, and religiously, we have been taught to care for our elderly or disabled parents in our homes until their last days. If we choose not to do so, it often evokes a sense of guilt. However, there are instances where we may find ourselves unable to provide the level of care they require.

There are many reasons why caring for a patient with Alzheimer's or other dementias is complicated. Some of these challenges include cognitive deterioration, caregiver burnout, the demands of 24/7 care, as well as the behavioral and physical changes that patients experience because of their disease, to name a few. These demands can significantly impact the caregiver's life. For instance, the patient may pose a danger to both themselves and others, and in some cases, they may even attempt to harm their own lives or the lives of their loved ones. Responsibly placing these patients in a long-term care home is an assertive decision because, with this decision, we are preventing harm to the caregiver, which could be irreparable.

In our personal experience, the idea of taking our father to a long-term care home was overwhelming and saddening. It stirred feelings of guilt and remorse, making us question, *'How could we relocate the best father in the world to a care home, distancing him from our lives?'* The mere thought of the potential pain and frustration stopped us from reaching a decision. However, fueled by love and the desire for our parents' well-being, we eventually mustered the courage to place him in a care home.

This decision would benefit our father, ensuring he received the quality care he deserved at a long-term center equipped with trained personnel specializing in Alzheimer's care.

Choosing to place a patient with Alzheimer's or other dementias in a long-term care center should not induce guilt. The crucial factor when deciding to relocate a patient is to supervise and ensure they receive the best possible care. As their children, witnessing the stability of our father receiving care in a trained center and observing the well-being of our mother, both physically and emotionally, freed us from guilt. We understood that we no longer had to feel guilty, as we were doing what was best for both of them.

XI. 10 RULES FOR BEING A GOOD CAREGIVER

In this section, we'll explore ten essential rules for being a compassionate and effective caregiver, empowering you with the knowledge and skills to navigate the challenges of Alzheimer's caregiving with grace and resilience.

1. ***Prioritize Physical Activity****: Establishing a regular exercise routine promotes both physical health and cognitive function.*

2. ***Embrace Nutritious Eating Habits****: A balanced diet rich in essential nutrients supports overall well-being and can enhance brain health.*

3. ***Eliminate Harmful Habits****: Avoiding smoking, excessive alcohol consumption, and high levels of stress helps maintain a supportive environment for both caregivers and patients.*

4. ***Recognize Mental Health****: Stay vigilant for signs of depression in yourself and your loved one, seeking support when needed to address emotional well-being.*

5. ***Acknowledge Limitations****: It's okay to admit when you're feeling overwhelmed. Saying "I CAN'T" and seeking help when experiencing burnout is crucial for sustainable caregiving.*

6. ***Prioritize Rest****: Ensuring an adequate amount of rest is essential for maintaining physical and mental health amidst the demands of caregiving.*

7. ***Foster Social Connections****: Cultivating a vibrant social life and engaging in enjoyable activities fosters a sense of fulfillment and helps prevent isolation.*

8. _**Maintain Order and Discipline**_: _Being disciplined and organized in caregiving tasks helps reduce stress and ensures effective management of responsibilities._

9. _**Attend to Health Needs**_: _Stay proactive in completing medical evaluations and preventive exams, adhering to medication regimens, and prioritizing you and your loved one's health._

10. _**Continuously Educate Yourself**_: _Commit to ongoing learning about Alzheimer's disease and caregiving strategies, empowering yourself with the knowledge to provide the best possible care._

XII. STATISTICS FOR CAREGIVERS <u>(AS OF 2023)</u>

1. *A very high% of caregivers quit their jobs so that they can take care of a patient with Alzheimer's.*

2. *Depression is the most common complication found in caregivers.[44]*

3. *An estimated 11 million people provide unpaid care to a patient with Alzheimer's or other dementias. [17]*

4. *Approximately 30% of caregivers for patients with Alzheimer's are above the age of 65.[17]*

5. *Approximately 2/3 of caregivers are women. [17]*

6. *66% of caregivers live with a person with dementia. [28]*

7. *Caregivers of patients diagnosed with Alzheimer's and other dementias carry a higher risk of suffering from depression.[44]*

8. *25% of caregivers are part of the sandwich generation, which simultaneously cares for their children and parents. [17]*

9. *70% of the costs produced by patients with Alzheimer's are paid by caregivers.[17]*

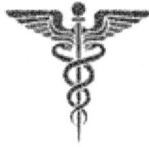

CHAPTER FIVE

Daily Activities: Recommendations for Better Care

I. INTRODUCTION

DAILY ACTIVITIES become disrupted as the disease progresses. Initially, the caregiver's intervention is minimal during the early stages; however, by the end of the disease, the patient's care depends 100% on the caregiver.

Alzheimer's disease presents in different stages, and patient care should be adjusted depending on their current stage. The caregiver's objectives should also change at every stage; during the mild stage, the goal is to supervise the patient's care with minimal intervention. In the moderate stage, the goal is to guide, manage, and promote independence for the patient. By the severe stage, the caregiver completes all necessities for them.

Educating ourselves provides us with the tools to adapt patient care based on the stage of their disease. It is essential to approach this with empathy and understand the frustration, sadness, and depression the patient may be experiencing. We must care for them with love, respect, and dignity. In the following pages, we will provide recommendations on how to navigate their daily activities.

II. BASIC DAILY ACTIVITIES

i. Clothing

✓ **Early Stage:** At this stage, the patient requires minimal help from the caregiver. The following recommendations for this stage also apply to older people who do not have Alzheimer's.

> ➤ Use anti-slip shoes.
> ➤ Size their shoes correctly.
> ➤ Use shoes with Velcro straps, never shoelaces.
> ➤ Never use pants or skirts that are too long, as this may cause the patient to fall.
> ➤ Do not wear tight clothes that may restrict their movement.
> ➤ Verify all clothing materials.

✓ **Moderate Stage:** At this point, the patient requires help to get dressed. Caregivers need to walk them through the steps of getting dressed, encouraging them to do it themselves.

> ➤ Use anti-slip shoes.
> ➤ Size their shoes correctly.
> ➤ Use shoes with Velcro straps, never shoelaces.
> ➤ Never use pants or skirts that are too long, as this may cause the patient to fall.
> ➤ Do not wear tight clothes that may restrict their movement.
> ➤ Verify all clothing materials.
> ➤ Do not wear pants with zippers.
> ➤ Use pants with elastic bands.
> ➤ If the patient prefers a specific type of clothing, purchase several or similar items.

✓ **Late Stage:** The patient is primarily bedridden or wheel-chair-bound, requiring complete assistance getting dressed.

> ➢ Always identify yourself when you are interacting with the patient.
> ➢ Smile!
> ➢ Complete tasks calmly.
> ➢ Explain all tasks to the patient.
> ➢ Use anti-slip shoes.
> ➢ Size their shoes correctly.
> ➢ Use shoes with Velcro straps, never shoelaces.
> ➢ Use comfortable cotton pajamas.
> ➢ Never use pants or skirts that are too long, as this may cause the patient to fall.
> ➢ Do not wear tight clothes that may restrict their movement.
> ➢ Verify all clothing materials.
> ➢ Do not wear pants with zippers.
> ➢ Use pants with elastic bands.

ii. *Dental Hygiene:* Dental hygiene is important to help prevent complications like cavities, gingivitis, tooth loss, and weight loss.

✓ **Early Stage:** The patient does not require assistance from their caregiver; however, they would benefit from verbal and written reminders.

> ➢ It is important to remind them to brush and floss their teeth daily.
> ➢ Remind them to take out their dentures and clean them every night.
> ➢ Always check their mouths for infections.
> ➢ Visit the dentist every six months.
> ➢ Use an electric toothbrush.
> ➢ Frequent reminders to use dental floss regularly.

✓ **Moderate Stage:** The patient requires assistance from their caregiver.

> Help them brush their teeth.
> Guide the patient daily; for example, go with them to the bathroom, find their toothbrush, hand it to them, add toothpaste, and guide them to do it themselves while the caregiver is present.[8]
> Rinse out the patient's mouth with water after each meal.
> Use either a kid's or soft-bristle toothbrush when brushing their teeth. Additionally, you may use kid's toothpaste.
> Remember to remove their dentures and put them away at night.
> While the patient's cognitive state allows it, visit the dentist every six months.

✓ **Late Stage:** During the late stage, many times, the patient's oral hygiene depends 100% on their caregiver.

> Once the patient is bedridden and is no longer responsive, the caregiver is responsible for rinsing their mouths with mouthwash and water.
> If possible, place the patient in a semi-sitting position.
> Always rinse their mouths with water.
> Use either a kid's or soft-bristle toothbrush when brushing their teeth. Additionally, you may use kid's toothpaste.
> Place the toothbrush gently into the individual's mouth, positioning it at a 45-degree angle. This angle allows for the massaging of gum tissue while effectively cleaning their teeth. 8
> Remove dentures if they are not needed.
> Use Alcohol-free, sensitive mouthwash.
> For unresponsive or ventilator-dependent patients, use cotton applicators soaked in mouthwash around their mouth to keep it clean. Always use another cotton applicator soaked in water afterward.
> Make sure the patient stays hydrated.
> Continuously monitor their oral mucosa for lesions, infections, etc., and notify their healthcare team.
> Ensure the lips of unconscious patients stay hydrated by applying moist cotton coated with Vaseline around them.

iii. Bathing

✓ **Early Stage:** The patient only requires written and verbal reminders.

✓ **Moderate Stage:** The caregiver must walk the patient through taking a shower and maintaining hygiene.

> ➤ Always introduce yourself when interacting with the patient.
> ➤ Prepare all necessary materials before starting: towel, shampoo, soap, water, etc.
> ➤ Always wash hands and use gloves.
> ➤ Protect the patient's privacy.
> ➤ Never leave them alone in the bathroom.
> ➤ Use a handheld showerhead.
> ➤ Support the patient by using a sturdy shower chair; this helps to reduce falls.[45]
> ➤ Start by testing the water with your fingers to ensure it is not too cold.
> ➤ Never point the shower head directly toward their heads; always point it toward their feet to ensure they're comfortable with the temperature. The patient may become fearful and anxious if the water is too cold.
> ➤ Follow this order when bathing: face, arms, underarms, thorax, abdomen, and genital area.
> ➤ Always wash off with water and dry off completely to avoid infections.
> ➤ Apply Vaseline to the patient's perineal area.
> ➤ Apply deodorant, lotion, and moisturizer to the patient's body.
> ➤ Change their bedsheets.
> ➤ Keep their nails trimmed.

✓ **Late Stage:** The patient spends most of their time bedridden. The task of bathing the patient relies entirely on their caregiver.

> ➤ Always introduce yourself when interacting with the patient.
> ➤ Routinely wash your hands and wear gloves.
> ➤ Always identify yourself when you are interacting with the patient.
> ➤ When bathing a bedridden patient, clean off their body from top to bottom. Start by washing their head.
> ➤ Keep up their oral hygiene. With a gauze pad, we swab the second finger of the hand.
> ➤ Use mouthwash or toothpaste around their mouth, lips, and tongue (minimum of two times).
> ➤ Use either a kid's or soft-bristle toothbrush when brushing their teeth. Additionally, you may use kid's toothpaste.
> ➤ Wash around their eyes and ears with a damp towel and soap. Wash and dry gently.
> ➤ Wash in the following order: arms, underarms, thorax, and abdomen. Wash and dry. Continue washing, starting with the legs. From the thighs to the feet on both sides, Wash and dry.
> ➤ Always wash from the cleanest area to the dirtiest area. Change used water and get new clean water if needed.
> ➤ Wash the back and the glutes. Wash and dry gently. Wash the perianal area from the front to the rear. Clean the area with disposable paper towels. Apply Vaseline to the perineal area when done.
> ➤ Whenever you have the patient by your side, take advantage of the opportunity and change their bedsheets. Place a pad, blanket, and diaper down to prevent the patient's skin from brushing against rough materials.
> ➤ Apply deodorant, lotion, and moisturizer to the patient's body.
> ➤ Protect the patient's privacy.
> ➤ Keep their nails trimmed.

iv. Shaving: The patient should use a razor only as long as their cognitive state allows. The caregiver must take over the task whenever they deem it unsafe for the patient to do so.

✓ **Early Stage**

➢ Remember to take care of the patient's beard and mustache. Leave them verbal and written reminders.
➢ Always remember to add any necessary material for beard hygiene to your grocery list.

✓ **Moderate Stage**

➢ Always identify yourself when interacting with the patient.
➢ Walk the patient through the steps of their beard hygiene routine.
➢ Try to encourage the patient to do it themselves.
➢ Leave verbal and written reminders for the patient.
➢ Often, the caregiver will need to guide the individual by applying shaving cream to their face and providing them with a razor while slowly mimicking the shaving movements to assess whether the patient can do it independently. The caregiver must assume that responsibility if the patient cannot perform the task.
➢ Constantly assess whether it is safe for the patient to have access to a razor.

✓ **Late Stage**

➢ Always Identify yourself when interacting with the patient.
➢ Walk them through the steps of their beard hygiene routine.
➢ If the patient is bedridden or cannot follow commands, then the caregiver is responsible for completing the routine.
➢ Always have all the necessary materials at hand before starting.

v. Hair Care

✓ **Early Stage:** The patient is entirely independent and can take care of their hair to their satisfaction.

✓ **<u>Moderate Stage:</u>** At this stage, the patient requires help caring for her hair. If it is possible, shorter hair is easier to manage.

> ➤ Always identify yourself when interacting with the patient. Walk them through the steps of what you're doing to keep them involved.
> ➤ Supervise them when they wash their hair and ensure they have everything they need to do it routinely.
> ➤ Consider transitioning to a shorter hairstyle. Shorter hair is often easier to manage and reduces the risk of tangles or knots.

✓ **<u>Severe Stage:</u>** During this stage, the caregiver assumes responsibility for maintaining the patient's hair. It is advisable to keep the hair short to facilitate easier management.

> ➤ Wash the patient's hair routinely. Use gentle products suitable for their hair type and scalp condition.
> ➤ Opt for a shorter hairstyle, this will make it easier to manage and maintain during this stage.
> ➤ While washing the patient's hair, provide gentle supervision and assistance as needed. Ensure they are comfortable throughout the process and have all necessary supplies readily available.

vi. *Eating:* The cognitive damage the patient suffers initially results in a loss of appetite and weight. Depending on the progression of the deterioration, the patient may have trouble swallowing and chewing. This continues until it reaches the final stage, where the patient stops eating altogether. You may initially lose your appetite and consequently lose weight for several reasons, including medications, behavioral alterations, hormonal changes, cognitive shifts, and others. As soon as you notice a loss of appetite, you must consult with your health team to identify the causes and work toward minimizing the problem.

✓ **Early Stage:** There are minimal changes in their eating habits.

> ➤ It is crucial to leave verbal and written reminders for the patient not to skip their meals, and lose weight as a result.
> ➤ Create weekly meal plans.
> ➤ It is important to promote a strict meal routine.

✓ **Moderate Stage:** The patient's diet starts to get affected due to their cognitive deterioration. The caregiver is now responsible for the preparation and supply of food.

> ➤ Add a touch of sweetness to meals (such as strawberries, grapes, or healthy sweeteners).
> ➤ Ensure that patients who wear glasses are wearing them while eating.
> ➤ Visit the dentist regularly to confirm good oral health.
> ➤ Provide healthy snacks every 2-3 hours.
> ➤ Turn off the television or radio during mealtime.
> ➤ Use the dining area for meals.
> ➤ Remove knives from the table.
> ➤ Ensure good lighting in the dining area.
> ➤ Supplement with vitamins and high calorie supplements if recommended by the healthcare team.[46]
> ➤ Offer finger foods.
> ➤ Serve small portions.
> ➤ Rinse mouth after meals.
> ➤ Establish consistent mealtime routines.
> ➤ Offer favorite foods.
> ➤ Purée food, if necessary.
> ➤ Limit food options on the plate to prevent confusion.
> ➤ Remove salt and pepper from the dining table.
> ➤ Avoid using disposable utensils, as the patient may chew and swallow them.
> ➤ Refrain from engaging in physical activities before meals.
> ➤ Avoid offering coffee.
> ➤ Refrain from offering dessert before the main meal.

✓ **Late Stage:** In the severe stage of Alzheimer's, patients become entirely reliant on their caregivers. They often face a loss of appetite, encounter difficulties with swallowing, and, as a result, experience weight loss.

> Constantly offer liquids.
> Verify the temperature of their food.
> Speak with their healthcare team and see if the patient would benefit from food thickener.
> Limit high-sodium items.
> Don't force the patient to eat if they don't want to. At this stage, the patient doesn't feel hunger or thirst.
> Offer foods that the patient prefers.
> Speak to their healthcare provider to see if changing their foods to purée consistency would benefit them.
> Avoid going out to restaurants.
> Offer food in small portions.
> Use spoons.
> Causes of dietary changes:

○ *Medications*
○ *Cognitive alterations memory loss*
○ *Clinical conditions*
○ *Depression*
○ *Poor Hygiene*
○ *Sensory changes*
○ *Vision problems*
○ *Loud environments*
○ *Taste loss*
○ *Difficulty swallowing and chewing*

> Notify your healthcare team if any of the following sound familiar:

○ *Unable to use utensils*
○ *Confuses designs on plates for real food*
○ *Confuses white bread for napkins; try to use whole wheat bread as a substitute*
○ *Difficulty grabbing food with hands*
○ *Holds food in their mouth*
○ *Spits out food*
○ *Difficulty swallowing*
○ *Chokes easily*

III. SAFETY IN THE HOME

Ensuring a safe and secure space becomes a foundational pillar of effective caregiving. In this chapter, we delve into essential strategies and precautions designed to safeguard the caregiver, the patient, and the home environment, fostering an atmosphere of security and tranquility amidst the complexities of dementia care.

i. *Early Stage*

- ✓ Keep all areas visible and well-lit.
- ✓ Assess all stairs and make structural changes if needed, i.e., adding a ramp.
- ✓ Place handrails in all hallways and bathrooms.
- ✓ Maintain hallways clutter-free to avoid any falls.
- ✓ Use night lights in the patient's bedroom.
- ✓ Always have a list of emergency contacts accessible to the patient.
- ✓ Place safety rails in any bathtubs.
- ✓ Keep a fire extinguisher in the kitchen.
- ✓ Avoid smoking near oxygen tanks, as this could be highly dangerous.
- ✓ Place anti-slip rugs in the bathroom.
- ✓ Make sure all medications are labeled and stored in a safe place.
- ✓ Label all cleaning products.
- ✓ Remove all firearms and consider returning any pertinent licenses.

ii. *Moderate Stage:* During this stage, the patient can no longer live alone for safety reasons and to avoid potential complications.

- ✓ Place handrails in the bathroom, including both showers and bathtubs.
- ✓ Place anti-slip rugs in the bathroom.
- ✓ Keep all areas visible and well-lit.

✓ Assess all areas of the house for any floor unevenness and make structural changes if needed.

✓ Evaluate if it is possible to place a ramp for future wheelchair needs.

✓ Verify all electric sockets are child-proofed.

✓ Avoid electric appliances in bathroom areas.

✓ The patient's bedroom and bathroom should be dimly lit throughout the night to help prevent falls.

✓ The patient requires assistance with bathing, food preparation, and driving. The caregiver must help take them to necessary appointments and complete any responsibilities outside the home.

✓ Ensure all medications are securely stored away from any areas accessible to the patient.

✓ Label all cleaning products.

✓ Avoid smoking near oxygen tanks, as this could be highly dangerous.

✓ Altogether, remove all the patients' firearms, as they should no longer have access to any hazardous weapons.

✓ Keep all doors closed at all times to help prevent the patient from running away and getting lost.

iii. *Late Stage:* To ensure the patient's safety, they should not live alone and require complete assistance from their caregiver.

✓ Place handrails in the bathroom, including both showers and bathtubs.

✓ Place anti-slip rugs in the bathroom.

✓ Keep all areas visible and well-lit.

✓ Assess all areas of the house for any floor unevenness and make structural changes if needed.

✓ Evaluate if it is possible to place a ramp for future wheelchair needs.

✓ Verify all electric sockets are child-proofed.

✓ Avoid electric appliances in bathroom areas.

✓ The patient's bedroom and bathroom should be dimly lit throughout the night to help prevent falls.

✓ Never leave the patient alone when bathing or in the kitchen.

✓ Bedridden patients with semi-electric beds should have the safety rails raised high at all times.

✓ Restrict patient access to medications.

✓ Altogether, remove all the patients' firearms and hand them to the relevant authorities.

✓ Discard medications according to the instructions labeled on them.

✓ Label all medications used, including those used explicitly for ulcer care.

IV. PAIN

Pain is a sensation that makes individuals feel uncomfortable changes in their bodies. It is challenging to manage pain in Alzheimer's patients because they often cannot communicate the type and intensity of pain they may be experiencing. As a result, these patients express their pain through behavioral changes.

It is our responsibility as caregivers to identify the signs of pain and immediately notify their healthcare team so that they can receive the necessary treatment. Educating ourselves will give us the tools to identify their pain, which is the first step in pain management.

i. **Early Stage:** The patient is currently independent and can verbalize their pain and explain its type.

> ✓ Check for signs of pain.
> ✓ Observe for behavioral changes that may indicate discomfort.
> ✓ Encourage the patient to communicate any discomfort or pain they may be experiencing, even if it seems minor.

ii. **Moderate Stage:** During this stage, the patient depends on the caregiver. They should be able to describe their pain, or at least express their pain through behavioral changes.

> ✓ Check for signs of pain.
> ✓ Consider using visual aids or pain scales to help the patient communicate their pain level more effectively.[47]
> ✓ Offer comfort measures such as gentle massage, positioning changes, or temperature regulation to ease any discomfort.

iii. Late Stage: The caregiver is fully responsible for completing all the patient's daily necessities.

 ✓ Check for signs of pain:

> ➤ Loss of appetite
> ➤ Painted facial expressions
> ➤ Pushes and shoves
> ➤ Sleep problems
> ➤ Grunts, moans, growls, cries, or constantly calls for the caregiver.
> ➤ Sadness, agitation, anger, or frowning
> ➤ Repeatedly touch a part of their body.
> ➤ Pleading eyes

iv. Tips to help decrease pain

✓If the patient is bedridden or wheelchair-bound, change the patient's position every 2 hours.

✓Move the patient little by little with slow and steady movements, especially with their joints.

✓Please do not do things rushed; it could hurt or cause the patient pain.

✓Observe to see if the patient has any ulcers, bruises, or lacerations that could cause them pain and immediately notify their healthcare team.

✓Go slowly when transferring the patient and ask for help if needed.

✓If you notice any signs of distress when moving the patient, immediately inform their healthcare team so that they may receive the necessary medications.

V. FALL RISK

Accidental falls are common in the elderly population; however, they are even more common in patients with Alzheimer's or other dementias. Unfortunately, these falls can be perilous and can lead to death. The reason these falls are so common is because of muscle weakness, psychiatric medication use, motor impairments, and attentional deficits, to mention a few.[48]

Patients diagnosed with Alzheimer's are predisposed to increased falls as a result of progressive cognitive deterioration, behavioral changes, and medication use.

i. Fall Prevention

✓ Early Stage

- Maintain all areas of the house well-lit and decluttered.
- Use safety rails around the house.
- Exercise a minimum of 25 minutes a day.
- Label everything.
- Avoid having unnecessary furniture clutter-ing up any areas.
- The patient's bedroom and bathroom should be dimly lit throughout the night to help prevent falls.
- If the patient suffers from incontinence, keep a portable toilet close to their bed.

✓ Moderate Stage

- Proper lighting in all areas around the house.
- Use safety rails around the house.
- Exercise as regularly as possible.
- Take advantage of non-pharmacological therapies that can be used to calm the patient.
- Prevent wandering.

> ➢ If the patient is incontinent, keep a portable toilet close to their bed.
> ➢ Keep the safety rails high up at all times if the patient uses a hospital bed.
> ➢ Verify their shoes and clothes are sized correctly.
> ➢ Keep all electric cables out of the patient's path.

✓ Late Stage

> ➢ Fall risk decreases.
> ➢ Proper lighting in the patient's room.
> ➢ Keep the safety rails high up at all times if the patient uses a hospital bed.
> ➢ If you are intervening with the patient, never leave them alone at any moment.
> ➢ Prevention always is the most critical step.

VI. SEXUALITY

As the patient progresses in their disease and their cognitive deterioration, they begin to suffer from sexual alterations, which manifest in different ways. This topic is very delicate, but the caregiver needs to be prepared so they know how to react correctly.

i. Sexual Alterations

- ✓ **Early Stage:** The most common sexual alteration patient's experience is apathy, which is usually caused by the depression and anxiety resulting from their diagnosis.[49]

    ➢ Consult your healthcare team.

- ✓ **Moderate Stage:** The patient may experience apathy, hypersexuality, inappropriate behaviors, and disinhibition.

    ➢ Consult your healthcare team.
    ➢ Avoid engaging in activities outside the house. Ensure the patient is supervised every moment they spend outdoors.
    ➢ Communicate with family members about the sexual disorders that your relative with Alzheimer's is experiencing and inform your health team to adjust their medications. This will help prevent uncomfortable situations arising from changes in sexuality.

- ✓ **Late Stage:** The patient no longer experiences any sexual alterations. They are most likely bedridden and are barely responsive to their environment.

    ➢ Consult your healthcare team.

ii. *Possible Types of Sexual Manifestation*

✓ **Sexual Apathy:** Absence of sexual interest.

✓ **Hypersexuality:** Exaggerated sexual interest with inappropriate actions toward inappropriate people such as their children, siblings, etc.

✓ **Dis-inhibited Behavior:** The patient may express their sexual desires publicly.

✓ **Inappropriate Behavior:** This behavior may be caused by memory loss, cognitive deterioration, or hallucinations, which can lead individuals to believe scenarios such as their significant other cheating or their child being the mistress.

If these behaviors are frequent, then consult your healthcare team for any recommendations they may have. Open communication with family members and healthcare providers is crucial in addressing and managing these delicate issues effectively. By staying informed and seeking appropriate interventions, caregivers can ensure the well-being and dignity of their loved ones throughout the progression of Alzheimer's disease.

VII. BOWEL & URINARY INCONTINENCE

In the realm of dementia caregiving, few challenges are as prevalent and impactful as urinary and fecal incontinence. The involuntary loss of bladder or bowel control can significantly disrupt the lives of individuals living with dementia, as well as those providing care. From the early stages of the disease, where incontinence may mimic age-related changes, to the later stages, where complete dependence on caregivers be-comes common, managing these issues effectively is crucial for maintaining dignity and quality of life. This guide will explore the causes, progression, and management strategies for both urinary and fecal incontinence, offering practical insights and support for caregivers navigating the complexities of dementia care.

i. ***Urinary Incontinence:*** The involuntary loss of urine where patients may leak or lose control of their urinary sphincter. There are different causes of urinary incontinence: pelvic muscle weakness, medications, prostate changes, dehydration, and neurological changes.[50] 60-70% of patients diagnosed with moderate or severe Alzheimer's are incontinent. [51]

    ✓ **Early Stage:** Incontinence at this stage presents the same way it does with any other individual of the same age.

        ➢ Visit the urologist annually.
        ➢ Complete UTI testing every six months.
        ➢ Stay hydrated.

    ✓ **Moderate Stage:** The patient is highly dependent on the caregiver, and they experience frequent incontinence, requiring the use of disposable diapers.

        ➢ Visit the urologist annually.
        ➢ Complete UTI testing every six months.
        ➢ Stay hydrated.

➢ Place pictures of the bathroom around so that the patient can locate it.
➢ Maintain a bathroom routine and use it every 2–3 hours.
➢ Limit the consumption of liquids before bedtime to avoid accidents. Always make sure that they are properly hydrated throughout the day.
➢ Take them to the bathroom before bedtime.

✓ **<u>Late Stage:</u>** The patient depends entirely on disposable diapers.

➢ Change diapers every two hours.
➢ Constantly evaluate the patient for signs of UTI
➢ Stay hydrated.
➢ Bathe the patient regularly, especially after they defecate.
➢ Keep genital areas clean at all times.
➢ Avoid using hygiene products that contain fragrances or alcohols.
➢ Avoid caffeine or alcohol.

ii. **Bowel Incontinence:** Fecal incontinence, also known as bowel incontinence, refers to the involuntary loss of bowel control, leading to the passage of fecal matter. It can be distressing for both individuals with dementia and their caregivers. Like urinary incontinence, fecal incontinence can have various causes, including muscle weakness, medications, dietary factors, and neurological changes.

✓ **Early Stage:** In the early stages of dementia, fecal incontinence may present similarly to individuals without cognitive impairment of the same age. However, caregivers should be vigilant for any signs of bowel control issues. Management strategies may include:

  ➢ Regular visits to a healthcare provider to address any underlying causes or concerns.
  ➢ Encouraging a balanced diet and adequate hydration.
  ➢ Establishing a regular toileting routine to promote bowel regularity.

✓ **Moderate Stage:** As dementia progresses to the moderate stage, fecal incontinence may become more frequent, requiring increased caregiver assistance.

  ➢ Regular visits to a healthcare provider for monitoring and management of bowel-related issues.
  ➢ Implement a toileting schedule, including frequent reminders for toileting.
  ➢ Provide easy access to the bathroom and maintain a consistent bathroom environment.
  ➢ Keep the patient hydrated.
  ➢ Observe any potential medication side effects, including those of laxatives and antibiotics.
  ➢ Avoid any dietary intolerances.
  ➢ Watch for loose stools and/or constipation.

✓ **Late Stage:** During this final stage of dementia, individuals may become entirely dependent on caregivers for toileting and hygiene needs.

> ➤ Observe any potential medication side effects, including those of laxatives and antibiotics.
> ➤ Changing soiled diapers as soon as possible to maintain skin integrity and prevent discomfort.
> ➤ Monitor for signs of bowel-related complications, such as constipation or impaction.
> ➤ Providing gentle and thorough perineal care after bowel movements to prevent skin irritation or infection.
> ➤ Avoid the use of fragranced or alcohol-based hygiene products, which can irritate sensitive skin.

VIII. PRESSURE ULCERS[52]

Pressure ulcers, commonly referred to as bedsores, are injuries caused by prolonged pressure and decreased circulation to an area of the skin. Prolonged obstruction of blood supply for a duration exceeding 2 to 3 hours initiates a process of skin deterioration, culminating in the formation of a painful lesion. Left unattended, such lesions have the potential to rupture, heightening the susceptibility to infection within the afflicted region.

Various types of ulcers exist, including diabetic ulcers, venous ulcers, those stemming from trauma, and pressure ulcers. Among patients diagnosed with Alzheimer's disease, pressure ulcers prevail as the most prevalent form of ulceration. These ulcers are categorized based on severity:

- ✓ **Grade I:** Intact skin with observable redness. The area may feel warm to the touch.

- ✓ **Grade II:** Open skin, with visible vesicles sores, or blisters. May experience significant pain.

- ✓ **Grade III:** Tissue loss, often with subcutaneous fat exposed.

- ✓ **Grade IV:** Extensive tissue loss, where fat, muscle, tendon, and even bone can be seen.

In the case of patients with Alzheimer's or other dementias in advanced stages of cognitive impairment, the patient cannot walk and spends more time sitting in a wheelchair or bedridden. This consequently causes pressure ulcers. These pressure ulcers form because the patient, unable to move, stays in the same position for over 2 hours, pressing the skin against the wheelchair or bed, which blocks blood supply to the area. Subsequently, the skin starts to develop ulcers.

i. *Early Stage:* The patient is independent and has no mobility problems; therefore, their risk for pressure ulcers is low.

- ✓ Constantly inspect skin.
- ✓ Inform their healthcare team of any abnormal changes.

ii. **Moderate Stage:** In this stage, the patient is at higher risk of developing pressure ulcers because they spend longer periods wheelchair-bound or bedridden. The patient also probably suffers from urinary incontinence and uses disposable diapers.

✓ Keep the area clean and dry.
✓ Check diapers every 2 hours, change as needed.
✓ Change the position of every wheelchair-bound patient every 2 hours.
✓ Use non-stick creams like Vaseline to help prevent ulcers.
✓ Use cotton bedsheets when possible.
✓ Regularly inspect the integrity of the patient's skin and notify their healthcare team if you see any changes.
✓ Place pillows or padding to minimize the risk of developing ulcers.
✓ Avoid using hygiene products that contain fragrances and alcohols.

iii. **Severe Stage:** The risk of developing ulcers is highest at this stage, as the patient is most likely bedridden and suffers from urinary incontinence.

✓ Prevention is key.
✓ Maintain the area clean and dry.
✓ Check diapers every 2 hours, change as needed.
✓ Change the position of every wheelchair-bound patient every 2 hours.
✓ Use non-stick creams like Vaseline to help prevent ulcers.
✓ Use cotton bedsheets when possible.
✓ Regularly inspect the integrity of the patient's skin and notify their healthcare team if you see any changes.
✓ Place pillows or padding to minimize the risk of developing ulcers.
✓ Avoid using hygiene products that contain fragrances and alcohols

IX. WANDERING

The patient, whether diagnosed with Alzheimer's or other forms of dementia, experiences increasing cognitive deterioration over time. Consequently, they become confused and disoriented in terms of time, place, and space. One of the common complications of this disorientation is wandering.

When the patient wanders, they walk aimlessly, searching for an exit or something unidentified. This is common among patients, and as caregivers, it is crucial to understand that it may serve as a way for the patient to communicate a need. This is when we use all the knowledge that we've learned to help identify their needs. While the reason behind their behavior may remain elusive, we can employ non-pharmacological therapy techniques to soothe the patient.

i. **Early Stage:** Cognitive deterioration and confusion are minimal at this stage. Wandering does not commonly occur during this stage.

> ✓ Supervise when the patient arrives and leaves the house for their safety.

ii. **Moderate Stage:** By this stage, the patient's cognitive deterioration has progressed, and they are confused, which makes the risk of wandering much higher.

> ✓ Implement safety plans.
> ✓ The house must be closed with a key at all times, and the caregiver must carry the key.
> ✓ The patient can never be left alone.
> ✓ Place an identifying bracelet on the patient, which includes their name and address, in case they get lost.

iii. Late Stage: There is a low risk of wandering at this stage, as the patient is most likely wheelchair-bound or bedridden. To avoid adverse outcomes, it is important to practice prevention.

✓ The patient can never be left alone.

iv. In Case of Elopement

✓ Look for the patient at home and in nearby surroundings.
✓ Notify the police.
✓ Notify all family members and neighbors so they can help look for the patient.
✓ Always have a recent picture available for identification purposes.
✓ Start a search for the patient, which includes places they frequented, streets, bodies of water, neighborhoods, etc.
✓ Call the nearest hospitals.

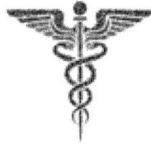

CHAPTER SIX

Communicating with Patients with Alzheimer's or other Dementias

I. INTRODUCTION

WHEN WE'RE born, our cry is how we communicate until we eventually develop the ability to speak and language becomes our primary method of communication. In patients diagnosed with Alzheimer's, communication and language are affected due to the damage to the brain and interruption of effective communication. The interruption of effective communication makes caring for the patient very difficult. Educating ourselves is our duty and responsibility to be able to effectively take care of a patient with Alzheimer's or other dementias.

In my practice, it is painful to listen when family members tell me how they try to correct the patient's behavior to bring them back to reality, as this action causes the patient's cognitive deterioration to accelerate.

"Go to their world; do not bring them to reality."

Communicating correctly helps us establish more effective communication patterns and diminishes stress, anger, and aggression. Establishing healthy communication results in an Alzheimer's patient who's happy and less mentally and physically exhausted.

II. WHAT IS COMMUNICATION?

Communication, the essence of human interaction, is the exchange of information between individuals. Effective communication necessitates both a sender and a receiver, manifesting through various channels, such as verbal language, non-verbal cues, visual aids, and written expression. These diverse forms facilitate understanding and connection between people.[53]

Under normal circumstances, communication relies on intricate neurological processes involving transmitting and interpreting information through neurons, receptors, and synapses. Disruptions of these processes can lead to communication inefficiencies. In conditions like Alzheimer's disease and other forms of dementia, such disruptions significantly impact communication, presenting challenges for both patients and caregivers. As the disease progresses, individuals may struggle to express themselves or comprehend others, leading to frustration and isolation.

Understanding the complexities of Alzheimer's and dementia is imperative for caregivers to develop effective communication strategies. Education about the disease equips caregivers with insights into patients' unique needs, enabling them to adapt communication methods accordingly. Beyond verbal interaction, non-verbal cues such as gestures, facial expressions, and body language play a crucial role in communicating with Alzheimer's patients. Visual aids and written communication also enhance understanding, particularly as verbal abilities decline in the later stages of the disease. By employing patience, empathy, and creativity, caregivers can navigate these challenges and improve the quality of life for patients and themselves.

III. HOW IS COMMUNICATION AFFECTED IN PATIENTS WITH ALZHEIMER'S

Alzheimer's disease impacts the brain in several ways, including neuronal death, disrupted neurotransmitter functions, and ultimately, interrupted synapses. This cascade of events leads to the eventual breakdown in communication within the brain, profoundly impacting individuals diagnosed with the disease. In addition to the physical changes occurring in the brain, Alzheimer's disease also affects the brain's ability to process sensory information effectively. Patients may experience difficulties interpreting auditory, visual, and tactile cues, further complicating communication. Because of these neurological changes, individuals with Alzheimer's often exhibit significant alterations in memory, language, and comprehension abilities, making traditional forms of communication ineffective.

Ultimately, navigating these communication challenges requires caregivers to be proactive, flexible, and understanding. By recognizing the impact of the disease on communication abilities and implementing appropriate strategies, caregivers can enhance the quality of life for individuals with Alzheimer's and foster meaningful connections despite the challenges they may face. In the following chapters, we will delve into specific techniques and strategies to communicate effectively with these patients, providing practical guidance for caregivers in navigating this aspect of care with confidence and compassion.

IV. UNDERSTANDING BEHAVIORAL CHANGES AND EFFECTIVE COMMUNICATION STRATEGIES FOR ALZHEIMER'S CARE

It's essential to understand when taking care of a patient with Alzheimer's that we need to educate ourselves and know that these behavioral changes are a form of communication. We should interpret and identify what exactly the patient is trying to communicate. These behavioral changes are not spiteful and are simply the patient's way of trying to signal their discomfort.

Identifying the message the patient is trying to send, processing it, and sending an appropriate response to the need they are trying to communicate. For us to be able to communicate effectively, we must Listen, Observe, Analyze, and Investigate.

For this to work, we need to know the patient. Know where they worked, their daily routine, medical conditions, relatives, preferences, culinary likes, religion, and everyday environment. Frequently, with alterations in behavior, the patient with Alzheimer's could be communicating some basic need to us but cannot verbalize it. It is essential to discern these basic needs consistently and address them; otherwise, the patient may become upset.

i. *Basic Needs*

✓ Hunger or thirst
✓ Feelings of sadness, boredom, nervousness, discomfort, or loneliness
✓ Sensation of feeling hot or cold
✓ Experiences pain
✓ Frequent urge to use the bathroom.
✓ Something is bothering them:

➢ Tight clothing
➢ Does not listen (Lost their headphones)

➢ Cannot see. (Lost their glass)

➢ Issues with eating (Dentures aren't fitted correctly)

ii. *Behavioral Disturbances as a Form of Communicating:*
The following are some examples of different ways that the patient may choose to communicate their needs:

✓ Agitation
✓ Screaming
✓ Kicking
✓ Cursing
✓ Scratching
✓ Biting
✓ Wandering
✓ Hostility
✓ Confusion
✓ Crying
✓ Humor changes
✓ Fear
✓ Trying to Elope
✓ Being sad, angry, or irritable

Identifying what the patient is trying to say is key. We should always remember, as caregivers, to take care of our loved ones with patience, empathy, compassion, sensitivity, and respect to allow our patients to be less frustrated, happier, and more cooperative.

V. AN ALZHEIMER PATIENT'S WORLD

"Go to their world; do not bring them to reality."

Understanding Alzheimer's disease and its effects on the brain is essential for caregivers tasked with providing care for diagnosed patients. Alzheimer's affects memory and impairs various cognitive functions, including perception, judgment, reasoning, analysis, and communication. Anosognosia, a common feature of Alzheimer's, further complicates the situation by rendering patients unaware of their illness. This lack of awareness can make it challenging for caregivers to provide appropriate care and support.

Anosognosia, the inability to recognize one's illness, is a hallmark of Alzheimer's disease. This phenomenon exacerbates the difficulty of caregiving, as patients may resist treatment or fail to understand the need for assistance. Caregivers must navigate this aspect of the disease with patience and empathy, recognizing that the patient's behavior is a manifestation of their cognitive impairment rather than deliberate defiance.

In the following sections, we will explore real-life scenarios to illustrate how Alzheimer's patients interact with their environment and how caregivers can adapt their communication approaches to better meet the needs of these individuals. By gaining insights into the unique challenges faced by Alzheimer's patients, caregivers can develop tailored strategies to enhance communication, foster meaningful connections, and provide compassionate care.

i. ***Scenario 1:*** The patient repeats repeatedly, *"I'm hungry,"* and can repeat it upwards of ten times. The patient is as unaware that they recently ate as they are of their cognitive deterioration. It's frustrating for caregivers and the healthcare team, as it's not true, but the patient believes it is.

✓ **Area Affected:** Memory

✓ **Incorrect Reaction:** Correcting the patient and telling them they have already eaten is wrong. When correcting the patient, they become frustrated with themselves for forgetting. The caregiver also feels frustrated because the patient is saying something wrong. In this case, the caregiver is in the wrong because the patient is hungry in their mind. They don't remember that they have not eaten, so we cannot bring them to our world. We need to go to their world and their reality, avoiding their frustration and anger in the process. This anger and frustration provoke depression, which can increase the progression of the patient's cognitive deterioration.

✓ **Correct Reaction:** Validate the patient's feelings and needs by avoiding corrections and instead acknowledging and being empathetic towards their hunger. Offer quick and healthy snacks while attempting to change the subject. It may be useful to help them complete a distracting task to redirect their focus.

ii. **Scenario 2:** Perception is a person's capacity to process information from a visuospatial perspective. The patient heads toward the front door, where they find a black welcome mat. They decide they do not want to stand on the welcome mat, and the caregiver tries to force them into the house.

✓ **Area Affected:** Perception

✓ **Incorrect Reaction:** Trying to force the patient to enter the home when they insist they do not want to. The patient is uncomfortable standing on the welcome mat; their perception is affected, making them believe it is a hole instead of a mat. The patient's response is most likely to get upset, scream, and shove because it is the only way they know how to communicate their fear.

✓ **Correct Reaction:** Respect the patient's perception and avoid forcing them to enter the home. Acknowledge their discomfort with the welcome mat and provide reassurance. Guide them gently away from the mat and prevent stepping on it to prevent frustration and anger. Engage in soothing conversation or distraction techniques to redirect their focus and reassure them of their safety. Alternatively, for a more straightforward solution, consider removing the carpet. Understanding the patient's perception and responding with empathy can prevent escalation of their fear and frustration.

iii. Scenario 3: It is important to recognize when a patient has communication problems due to their memory and language being affected. The patient gets agitated, screams, wanders, and has other behavioral changes that indicate that the patient is trying to communicate a need.

✓ **Area Affected:** Communication

✓ **Incorrect Reaction:** The caregiver attempts to reason with the patient, questioning them with statements such as, *"Why are you upset? What's wrong with you? Come sit here! And stay put!"* However, the caregiver often becomes frustrated, as the patient's reaction is likely adverse. The patient may experience heightened anger and exhaustion, even resorting to attacking the caregiver in response to feeling misunderstood.

✓ **Correct Reaction:** Step away from engaging the patient in reasoning or questioning and instead focus on providing reassurance and comfort. Approach the patient calmly, using gentle and soothing tones. Offer simple statements such as, *"I understand you're upset. Let's find a solution together!"* Redirect the patient's attention to a different activity or area to help alleviate their agitation. It's important for the caregiver to remain patient and understanding, avoiding any confrontational language or actions that may escalate the situation further.

iv. Scenario 4: The patient attempts to *"elope"* from their house every day around 3 pm because, in their daily life, they used to pick up their children from school at that time. So, now, around the same time every day, they try to leave the house because, in their world, they're trying to pick up their children like they used to.

✓ **Area Affected:** Patients *"freedom"*

✓ **Incorrect Reaction:** Once we have identified that the patient is trying to elope, we start trying to address the issue without analyzing the situation. We try to do so by arguing with and explaining to the patient why they cannot elope. We then order the patient to stay away from the door, which leaves them angry, frustrated, and confused about why they cannot pick up their children. Imagine how you would feel as a mother if you were prevented from picking up your children from school.

✓ **Correct Reaction:** Once you have identified the patient's desire to elope, explore the reasons behind it. Familiarize yourself with the patient, their likes, religion, occupation, and daily activities to gain insight. Perhaps the patient feels like they're waiting for someone or has pending tasks, which may make them feel the need to leave the house. The following scenario describes an appropriate way to both calm and distract the patient away from the door.

➢ *Patient: "I need to pick up my children from school."*
➢ *Caregiver: "Do not worry, Mr. or Mrs. _____, your partner is picking up the kids today."*

v. ***Scenario 5:*** The patient is wheelchair bound and is constantly sad and crying while they refuse to eat or leave their beds. Despite attempts from caregivers to encourage movement and eating, the patient's sadness persists, causing visible distress and a strong refusal to participate in anything beyond staying in bed.

✓ **Area Affected:** Patient happiness.

✓ **Incorrect Reaction:** You immediately approach the patient and explain the importance of getting up. You then proceed to forcefully insist they eat and bring them food, which causes the patient to kick, scream, and throw the food on the floor.

✓ **Correct Reaction:** Avoid attempting to reason with the patient, who may be experiencing deep sadness and reluctance to leave their bed. Instead, offer genuine empathy and support by approaching them with a smile and a comforting hug. Express your willingness to assist them without imposing any immediate expectations. Take the time to observe, analyze, and investigate the underlying reasons for their behavior, considering factors such as homesickness or emotional distress. Tailor your approach to each patient's individual needs, prioritizing their emotional well-being and comfort.

VI. COMMUNICATION TECHNIQUES WITH AN ALZHEIMER'S PATIENT

Within the following pages, you will find a collection of scenarios depicting interactions with patients diagnosed with Alzheimer's disease. These scenarios aim to provide caregivers with valuable insights into the challenges they may encounter while caring for individuals with Alzheimer's and other forms of dementia. Each scenario is carefully crafted to illustrate everyday situations caregivers may face, accompanied by an explanation of the underlying cognitive processes influencing the patient's behavior.

By delving into these scenarios, caregivers can gain a deeper understanding of the complex nature of Alzheimer's disease and learn effective strategies for navigating the unique needs and behaviors of their loved ones or patients.

✓ Smile!
✓ Use simple language
✓ Identify yourself:
  ➢ *"Hello, I'm ___, your daughter/son"!*
✓ Do not reprimand or shame them.
✓ Ask simple questions:
  ➢ *"Are you cold?"*
  ➢ *"Would you like to go out?"*
✓ Do not talk about them as if they're not there.
✓ Do not contradict or argue with them.
✓ Instead of saying, *"No, you can't"*, say, *"Yes, we can do it together."*
✓ NEVER SAY: *"Don't you remember?"*
✓ Do not say: *"...I told you so."* Simply repeat it as many times as necessary.

Scenario I: Always Smile

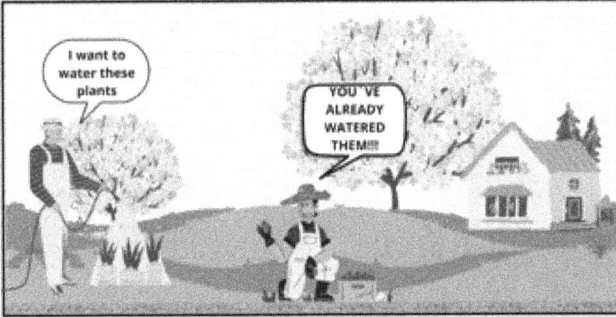

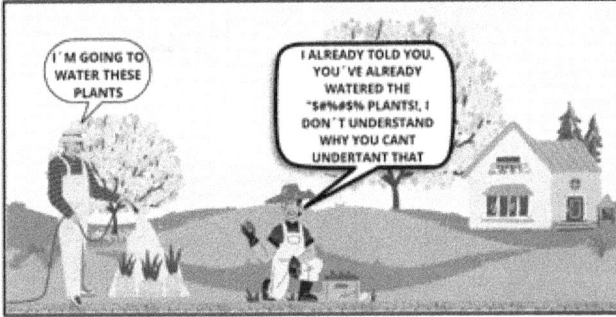

Smile, patients with Alzheimer's respond in the same way they are treated.

If you smile and speak softly, the patient will smile.

If you talk to them angrily, they will respond angrily.

Scenario II: Avoid Sarcasm

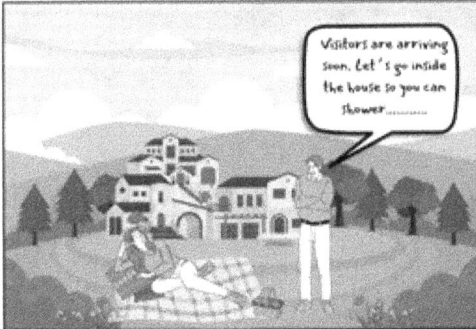

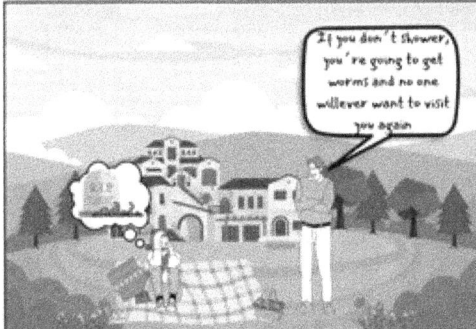

Patients with Alzheimer's and other dementias, are unable to understand sarcasm because they confuse it with reality.

Scenario III: Identify Yourself

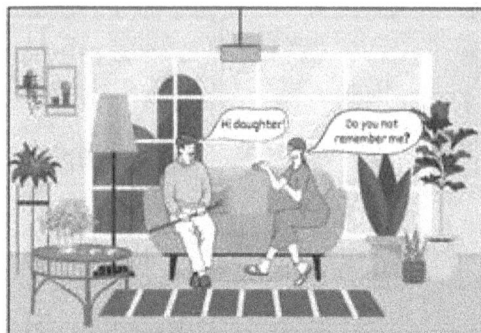

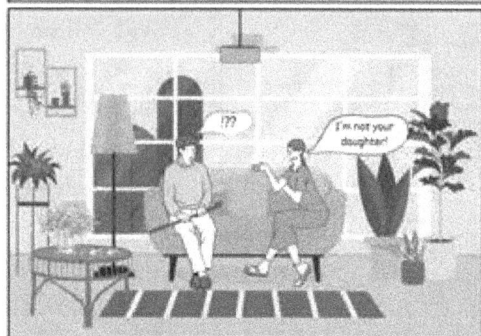

Scenario IV: Shame-Free Care

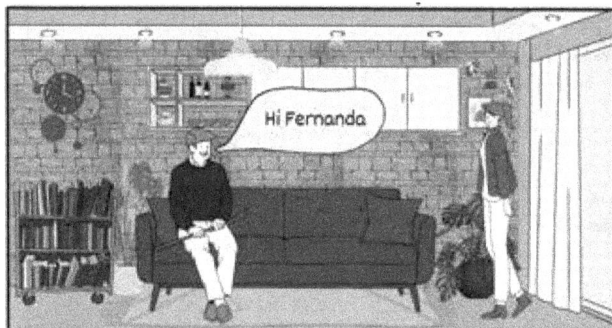

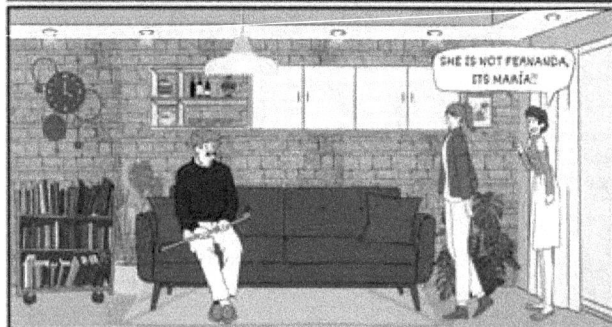

Scenario V: Simple Questions

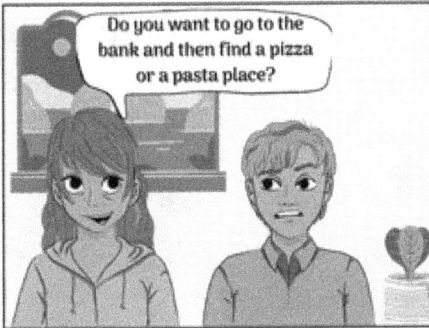

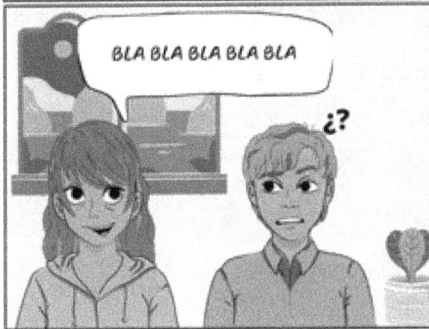

Don't ask long questions, be concise and ask simple questions like:

Are you cold?
Would you like to go out?
Do you want to eat?

Asking short questions can help prevent the patient from feeling overwhelmed and allow them to make quicker decisions.

Scenario VI: Be Respectful

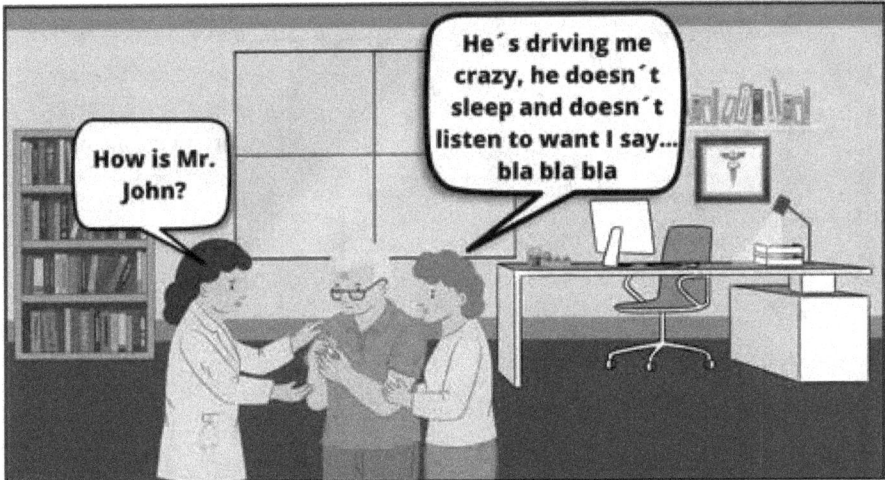

Its important to communicate effectively with the patients healthcare team. Communicate any concerns you may have in the patient's abscence.

Scenario VII: Avoid Arguments

Scenario VIII: Include Them

When completing an important task, it is important to give the patient detailed instructions on how to do so. As a caregiver, it is not healthy for you to do it all by yourself. It can be more helpful to calmly get their attention and try to involve them in the task. Doing so in a loving way, can help the patient feel included and useful.

Scenario IX: Never Say "Do You Not Remember"

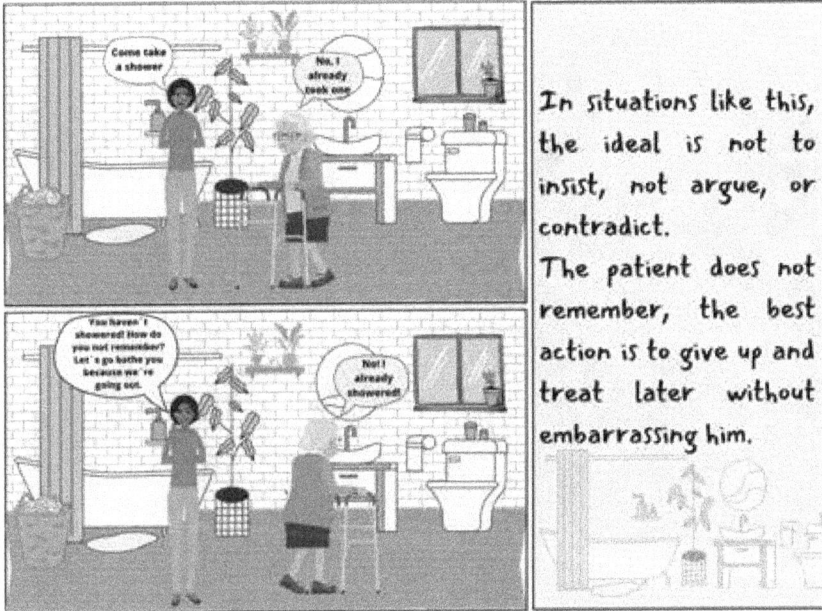

In situations like this, the ideal is not to insist, not argue, or contradict.
The patient does not remember, the best action is to give up and treat later without embarrassing him.

Scenario X: Never Say "I Told You So"

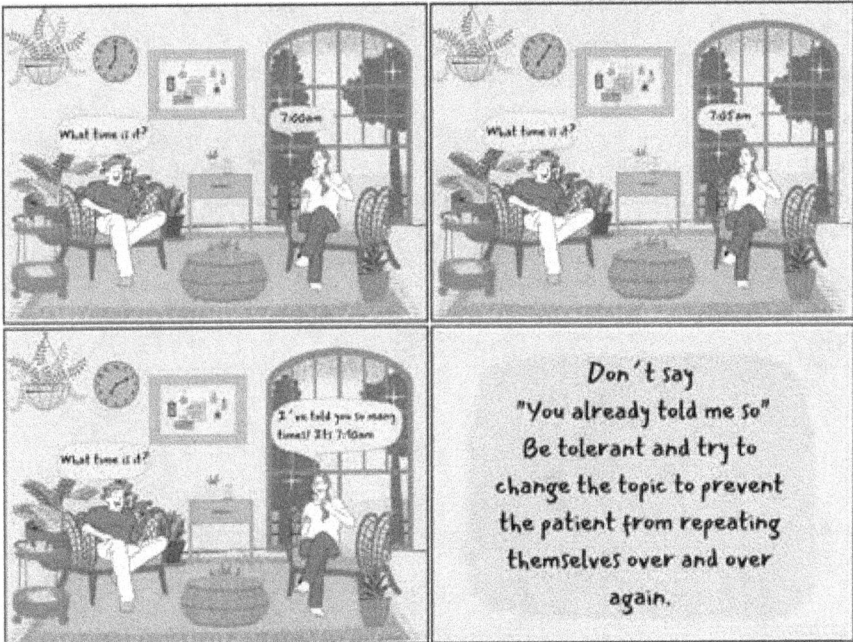

Don't say "You already told me so" Be tolerant and try to change the topic to prevent the patient from repeating themselves over and over again.

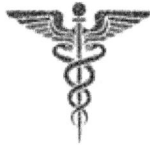

CHAPTER SEVEN

Legal & Financial Planning

I. INTRODUCTION

PLANNING FOR the future should be a priority for everyone. However, in the case of a patient with Alzheimer's, it is essential to avoid complications as cognitive impairment progresses and the patient becomes incapacitated. Throughout the book, we have emphasized the importance of diagnosing Alzheimer's as early as possible so that the patient can receive adequate treatment and plan their financial and legal future.

The result of financial and legal planning will be the peace of mind of knowing that their care will not be impacted by a lack of economic resources or by not having made financial arrangements. There is also satisfaction in knowing that their decisions will be respected per their wishes. It is important to point out that legal and financial planning should comply with the laws of their country and its governmental institutions.

The goal is to protect yourself, legally and financially, in the event of a disability.

II.RECOMMENDATIONS FOR PLANNING YOUR LEGAL AND FINANCIAL FUTURE

- ✓ Speak with a person you trust or relatives regarding your wish to plan your legal and financial future.
- ✓ Hire a lawyer you trust and ask them for legal advice according to the laws of your country.
- ✓ Assign legal guardianship to the person you wish to be responsible for following through with your wishes. Ask that person if they accept the responsibility.
- ✓ Allow the above person access to complete transactions at any financial institution in your name in the case of disability.
- ✓ Actualize and organize all legal documents, including wills, insurances, bank accounts, life insurance, assets, and advance directives. Notify your person of trust or your legal guardian of the documents' location.
- ✓ Set aside an adequate amount of money designated for your care in the case of disability to assist your legal guardian in providing for you.
- ✓ Redact your will.
- ✓ Redact your advanced directives.

III. THE WILL

The will is a legal document created by a person of legal age and capacity, wherein they express their wishes regarding the distribution of assets and rights after their death. It must be in writing, include a date, and preferably be prepared in front of a lawyer. It's important to point out that the person must have legal capacity for a will to be valid. This is why, in patients with Alzheimer's, the will must be executed in the initial stages of the disease.

In the will, all assets, money, and insurance must be listed, along with how they will be distributed in the event of the person's death. Writing a will has several benefits, including avoiding problems among family members, ensuring assets are distributed according to one's wishes, and minimizing court intervention. The person creating the will must decide on the executor (the person in charge of enforcing the will).

Once the will is drafted, it's not a document to be forgotten. It is not recommended for patients with Alzheimer's or other dementias to continue changing their will as their condition progresses. Keeping a will ensures that the individual's wishes are respected and reduces the likelihood of disputes or legal complications down the line.

IV. FINANCIAL PLANNING

Financial planning involves setting a budget, determining how debts will be paid, designating a person authorized to intervene in checking bank accounts or savings, and selecting a trusted individual to prevent financial abuse in case of disability.[54] It is crucial to start planning early, as soon as the diagnosis is made, to ensure that individuals with Alzheimer's maintain legal capacity at the time of planning.

Planning for the future will provide peace of mind, assuring that expenses will be covered and that care will not be disrupted. Consult with your banking institution and its financial advisors to seek assistance and monitor for fraudulent activities.

It's imperative to explore various financial options and resources available for individuals with Alzheimer's and their caregivers. This might include looking into long-term care insurance, Medicaid eligibility, and veteran benefits. Additionally, establishing a durable power of attorney, which will be discussed in the following section, can facilitate the management of financial affairs when the individual with dementia can no longer make sound decisions. Creating a comprehensive estate plan, including a will or trust, can also help protect assets and ensure that the individual's wishes are carried out according to their preferences. Financial planning is about managing current expenses and safeguarding assets for the future, providing a sense of security and stability during what can be a challenging time.

V. POWER OF ATTORNEY

A power of attorney is a legal document created by a person of legal age and capacity. It is executed in the presence of a lawyer. In the document, the person seeking a power of attorney designates a trusted individual to decide on their behalf in the event of disability. If the person who granted the power of attorney passes away, the authority conferred by the document becomes invalid.

In the case of patients with Alzheimer's, the legal power is determined in the initial stages of the disease as long as the patient retains legal capacity. The authority may be subject to other legal procedures if the patient loses legal capacity. It is crucial to consistently seek advice from your legal representatives and draft documents per the laws of your country.

Having a power of attorney early on allows for a smoother transition of decision-making authority to a trusted individual, ensuring that the patient's best interests are upheld, and their wishes are respected. Without a power of attorney, the legal process becomes more complex and time-consuming, often resulting in decisions made by the court rather than those who intimately understand the patient's needs and preferences. Therefore, caregivers are strongly encouraged to engage with legal professionals to establish a power of attorney and navigate the intricacies of legal and financial planning tailored to their specific circumstances and jurisdiction.

VI. ADVANCED DIRECTIVES

Advanced directives are medical decisions stipulated in a legal document, as explained in Chapter 3. This legal document is prepared by a person of legal age and capacity, establishing their last wishes according to their medical decisions.

Advanced directives are crucial in ensuring that your medical wishes are honored even if you cannot communicate them yourself. By clearly outlining your preferences regarding medical treatments, interventions, and end-of-life care, you provide invaluable guidance to your loved ones and healthcare providers. These directives can include instructions on life-sustaining measures, resuscitation preferences, and the designation of a healthcare proxy to make decisions on your behalf.

Taking proactive steps to establish and communicate your wishes can ease stress and uncertainty for your caregivers and ensure that your healthcare decisions align with your values and beliefs. When filing your advanced directives, the crucial aspect is ensuring that, in case of incapacity, the provisions you have arranged will prevent discrepancies among family members who may need to make decisions on your behalf.

VII. LEGAL DOCUMENTS

Legal documents legally establish possession of property, declarations, rights, obligations, etc. These documents protect people's rights. Some examples include:

- ✓ Birth certificate
- ✓ Marriage certificate
- ✓ Social security card
- ✓ Advanced directives
- ✓ Property titles
- ✓ Wills
- ✓ Leases & Loans
- ✓ Legal guardianship
- ✓ Bank accounts
- ✓ Life insurances
- ✓ Others

In the realm of caregiving for individuals with Alzheimer's and other dementias, organizing and safeguarding legal documents is paramount. These documents establish ownership and rights and serve as crucial tools for ensuring the well-being and protection of the individual and their assets. It's imperative to maintain these documents in a designated safe location accessible to trusted individuals, especially the legal guardian, in case of incapacitation or emergency. Caregivers should prioritize establishing clear communication channels regarding the location and significance of these documents to facilitate efficient decision-making and legal processes when needed.

VIII. LEGAL GUARDIANSHIP

Legal guardianship in the context of Alzheimer's or other forms of dementia is a critical aspect of caregiving and long-term planning. When an individual's cognitive abilities decline to the point of incapacitation, the appointment of a legal guardian becomes necessary to ensure their well-being and protect their interests.

The legal guardian, as designated by the court, assumes a weighty responsibility. They are entrusted with making essential legal and medical decisions on behalf of the incapacitated individual. These decisions may range from healthcare choices to financial matters, all aimed at responsibly providing the best possible care and managing assets. This includes overseeing day-to-day needs, medical treatment, housing arrangements, and end-of-life care. Moreover, the legal guardian must navigate complex financial transactions, ensuring that the incapacitated person's assets are managed sensibly and their financial affairs are handled meticulously.

Legal guardianship serves as a safeguard against potential exploitation and ensures that the person with dementia receives the necessary care and protection. However, it also underscores the importance of proactive planning. By arranging legal documents such as powers of attorney and advanced directives while still of sound mind, individuals can help avoid the need for court intervention later on.

It's essential to recognize that legal guardianship laws and procedures vary from one country to another. Caregivers and family members must familiarize themselves with their jurisdiction's specific legal requirements and processes. This knowledge empowers them to navigate the legal system effectively and advocate for the best interests of their loved ones.

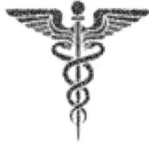

CHAPTER EIGHT

Alzheimer's & Kids

I. INTRODUCTION

THE DIAGNOSIS of a family member with Alzheimer's impacts everyone, and family members, including children, are no exception. Nostalgia comes to mind as I develop this topic; my children were little when my father was diagnosed with Alzheimer's. Questions arose in their young minds: *why didn't their grandfather remember them? Why did he act strangely? Why didn't he play with them anymore?* These were just a few of the many questions I was responsible for answering.

Children, as integral parts of our family, have the right to understand what Alzheimer's disease is, along with the future symptoms, explained in terms appropriate to their age. This approach helps involve them as active members of the family. Educating children about the disease, its different stages, symptoms, and progression will help prevent feelings of fear and anxiety.

It becomes the responsibility of the children's parents or guardians to decide whether to explain the family member's medical condition to them and how explicit they should be. This decision depends on the child's relationship with the diagnosed patient. If the child has infrequent direct contact with the family member, being overly explicit may not be necessary, as they may not witness any cognitive damage or different behavioral manifestations. On the contrary, if the child interacts with the relative more frequently, explaining the symptoms, disease progression, and possible behavioral changes becomes essential.

The decision on when, how, and why to explain Alzheimer's or other dementias to children will always be a matter of parental discretion and responsibility.

II. THE RIGHT AGE TO EXPLAIN ALZHEIMER'S TO KIDS

There is no specific age to explain Alzheimer's disease to a child; what matters is identifying the appropriate moment to discuss the disease, its symptoms, stages, and, most importantly, the progression of the disease and its complications.

The complexity of how we explain it depends on the child's age and ability to learn and understand the disease. The opportune moment arises when the child starts asking questions, such as:

✓ *"Why does your family member behave like this?"*

✓ *"Why doesn't your family member recognize others?"*

✓ *"Why doesn't their family member play with them?"*

✓ *"Why does your family member become aggressive?"*

The child will comprehend that the behaviors exhibited by a person with Alzheimer's are complications of the disease, and they will understand that these changes are not intentional, nor are they a result of their grandparent being inherently bad.

Recent statistics reveal that many caregivers belong to the *'sandwich'* generation, meaning they are simultaneously caring for children and a family member with Alzheimer's.[55] It is our responsibility to explain to the child what is happening so that the child's emotional stability is not adversely affected by the illness of their family member.

III. HOW TO EXPLAIN ALZHEIMER'S

The vocabulary and level of explicitness we use to discuss Alzheimer's disease with children depend on their age, attention, and interest in the topic. Explain simply that Alzheimer's is a brain disease; the brain is a part of the human body, and its primary function is to control actions, thoughts, judgment, and memory, among other things.

In the case of a patient with Alzheimer's, explain to the child that the brain is sick, causing the person to behave differently, forget who they are, forget to play, and possibly become aggressive. While the patient may not remember us, we remember them and their love. It's crucial to teach children that these situations are part of life, and the important thing is to support our family by providing love and practicing tolerance.

Children may have many questions for which we do not have all the answers, but our attitude and education on the subject will equip us to explain it to the child, avoiding fear and anxiety. Most importantly, this approach will foster empathy toward the loved one and promote respect, love, and tolerance in the child.

IV. A CHILD'S ATTITUDE TOWARD ALZHEIMER'S DISEASE

"Attitude" is the way we react to a situation. It is normal for us to feel sad, frustrated, and in pain, but we must always assume responsibility. If we decide to care for a family member with Alzheimer's, we must do it with love, respect, and dignity, maintaining an attitude of empathy. As caregivers of a family member with Alzheimer's or other dementias, we must avoid any form of abuse. It is important to recognize symptoms of burnout in ourselves and evaluate whether taking care of our family members is the best decision to prevent setting a negative example for our children.

The main reason for writing this guide is to impact families with a member suffering from Alzheimer's or other dementias. I aim to guide them in seeking help if necessary and to avoid projecting feelings of frustration and depression onto children, as it could negatively impact their lives. We must use this situation to help our children understand it is okay to feel sad, but our relative with Alzheimer's deserves and needs all our love and the best possible care, especially love. Explain to children that these feelings should not influence how we care for our family members with Alzheimer's.

Emotionally, we are responsible for the stability of our children. Therefore, we must provide them with tools to face not only the illness of our family members but also any other situation. As caregivers, we set an example of how to face and react to a patient's illness with Alzheimer's. If we respond with frustration, depression, or distress, children will likely mirror these emotions. Children reflect our attitudes, so let's be mindful of them.

V. EDUCATE CHILDREN TO COMMUNICATE EFFECTIVELY WITH AN ALZHEIMER'S PATIENT.

Communicating with a loved one affected by Alzheimer's or another form of dementia can be challenging. Still, it's a skill that children can learn to navigate with patience and understanding. In this chapter, we'll explore how to teach children effective communication strategies tailored to the unique needs of individuals with Alzheimer's. Through a series of scenarios, we'll illustrate correct and incorrect responses, empowering children with the knowledge and tools to engage with their family members meaningfully and respectfully. By equipping children with these essential communication skills, we can foster deeper connections and enhance the patient's and their families' quality of life.

- ✓ Respect all patients.
- ✓ Smile!
- ✓ Never contradict them; call their caregiver if necessary.
- ✓ Be kind and cordial when speaking to them.
- ✓ Always identify yourself:
  - ➢ *"Hi grandpa, I´m your ____ Granddaughter!"*
- ✓ Speak about topics they enjoy.
- ✓ Never make fun of them or embarrass them.
- ✓ Never say: *"Grandpa! I already told you that."*

VI. HOW CHILDREN CAN HELP CARE FOR A PATIENT WITH ALZHEIMER'S.

Children can take part in caring for our patients with Alzheimer's in various ways. It is crucial to emphasize that when discussing how children can help care for a family member with Alzheimer's, they should NEVER BE LEFT ALONE with the patient. However, children can still contribute significantly by alerting us in emergencies, entertaining the patient, and assisting with simple tasks such as handwashing, among other activities. Below are some scenarios illustrating how children can help care for a patient with Alzheimer's or other dementias.

Scenario I

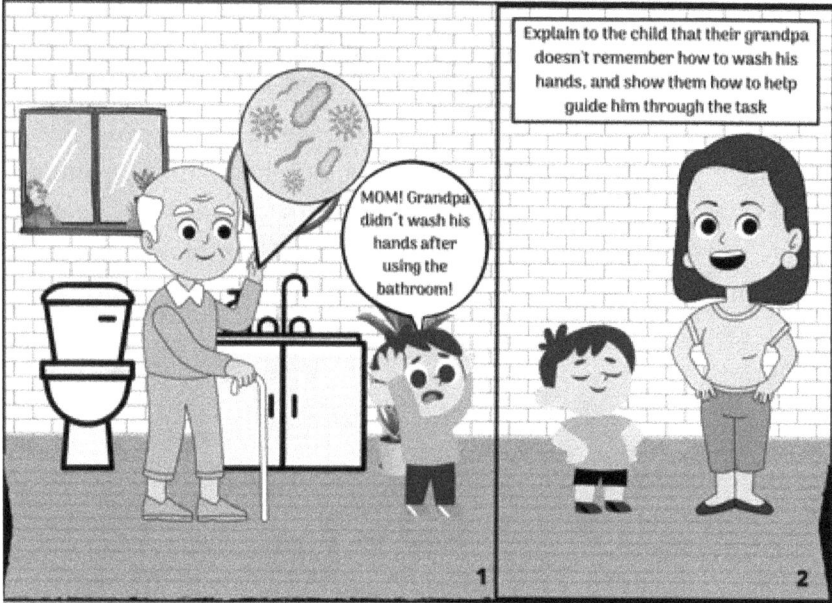

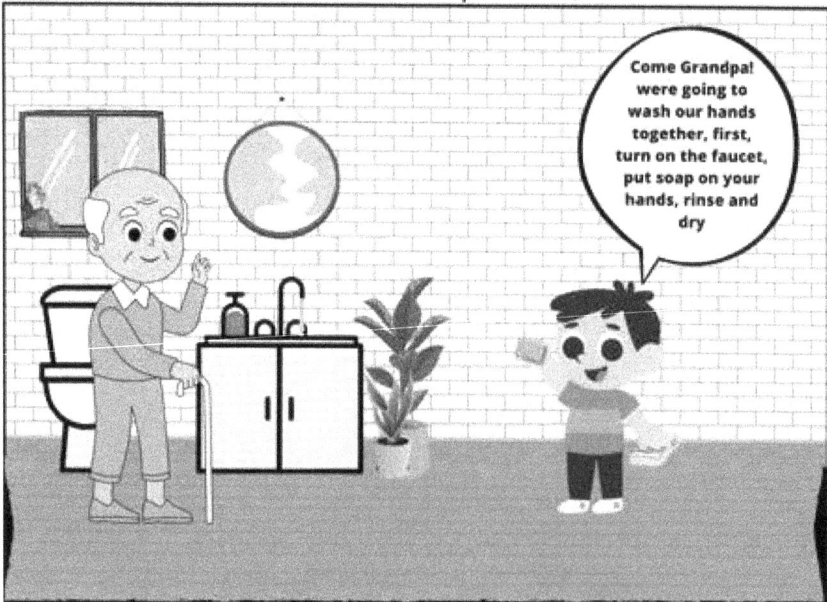

Scenario II

Incorrect Response

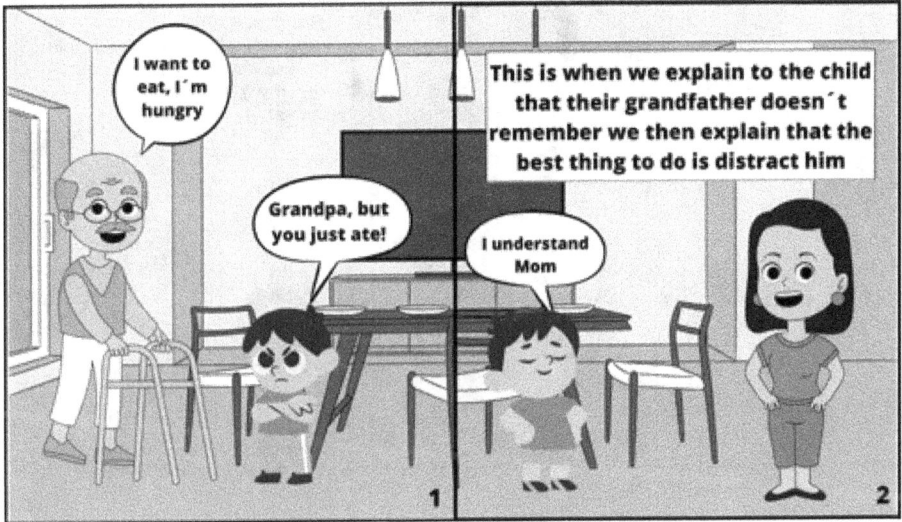

Correct Response

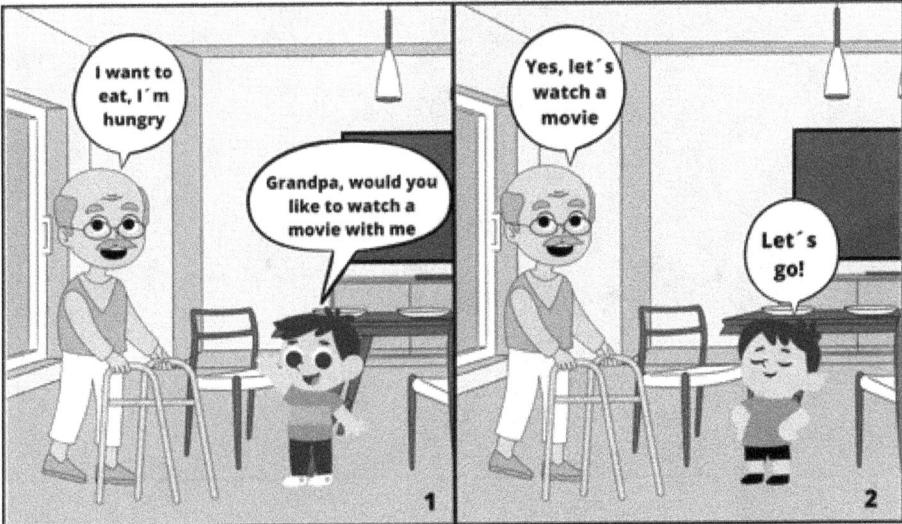

Scenario III

Incorrect Response

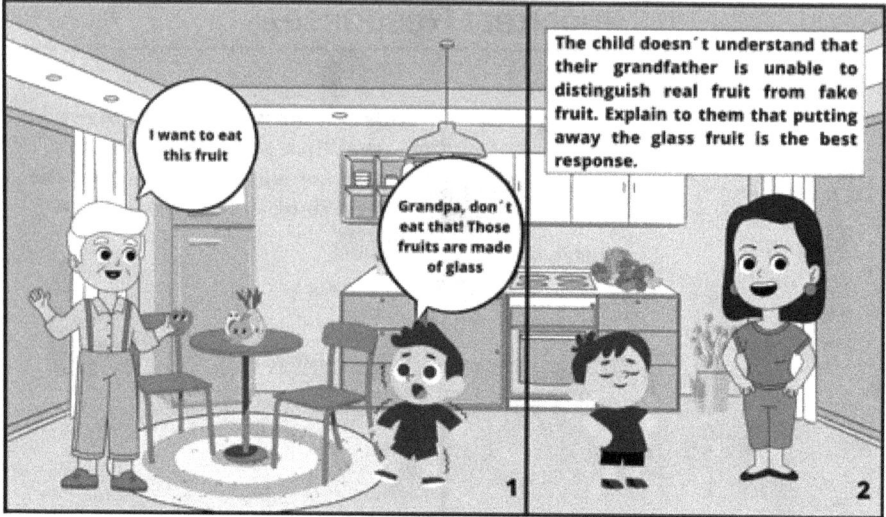

Correct Response

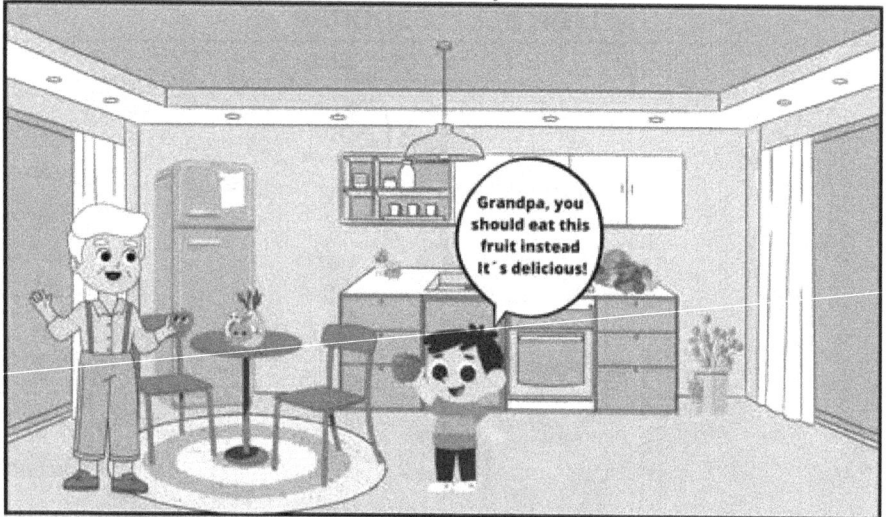

Scenario IV

Incorrect Response

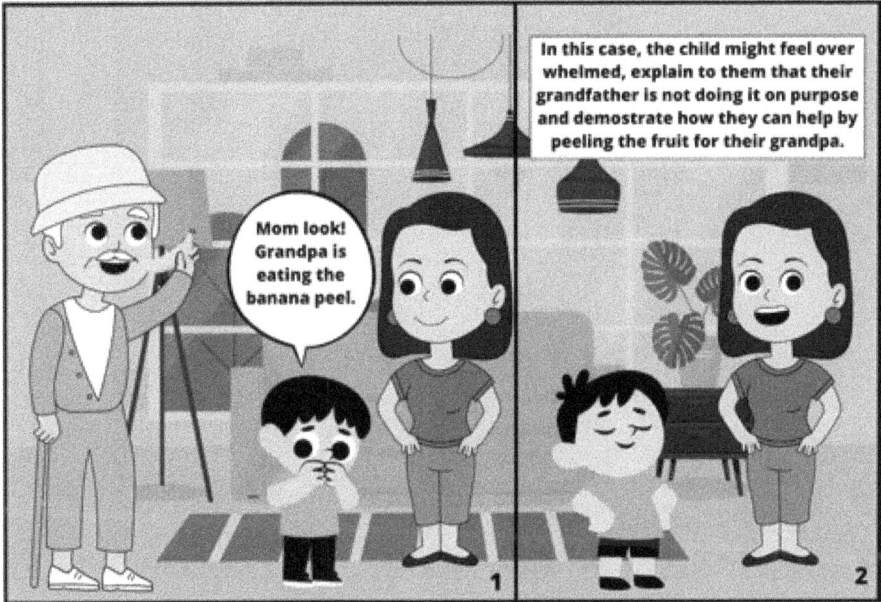

Correct Response

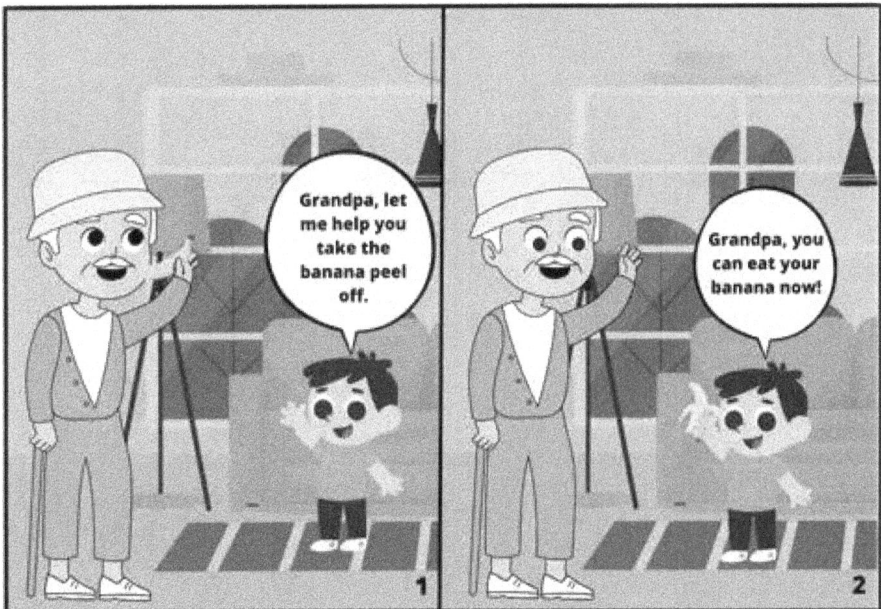

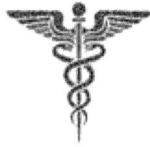

CHAPTER NINE

Recompense

IN GRATITUDE FOR the perfect and pure love that our father provided us, we reciprocated by providing him with excellent care. This allowed us to express our appreciation for his love, effort, and dedication in caring for us. Caring for a patient with Alzheimer's or other dementias is not a simple task, just as raising a child is not. However, love guides us, and with guidance, education, and a good team, we can excel in our responsibilities as caregivers. The effort, dedication, and love we invest in caring for our family member with Alzheimer's or other dementias will be one of the most rewarding experiences in our lives.

When we embark on the journey of caregiving for a loved one with Alzheimer's or dementia, it's essential to understand that it's not just about fulfilling a duty or obligation. It's about honoring the person they were before the disease took its toll and recognizing their continued worth and dignity. Every moment spent caring for them is an act of compassion and respect, a testament to the bond between us and our loved ones. Moreover, caregiving is not one-sided; it's a reciprocal relationship that enriches the caregiver and the recipient. While it may seem like a daunting task, with its challenges and uncertainties, it also presents countless opportunities for growth, resilience, and personal fulfillment. As caregivers, we learn patience, empathy, and selflessness, qualities that benefit us in our role and extend to other areas of our lives.

In addition to the emotional rewards, caregiving can lead to personal growth and transformation. It challenges us to step outside our comfort zones, confront our fears and limitations, and tap into reservoirs of strength and resilience we never knew we had. It teaches us to appreciate life's simple joys and find beauty and meaning in moments of vulnerability and uncertainty.

Ultimately, recompense in caregiving is about finding purpose and ful-fillment in the act of giving and receiving love unconditionally. It's about embracing the journey with an open heart and a willingness to learn and grow every step of the way. As we navigate the complexities of Alzheimer's and dementia care, let us remember that the greatest reward lies not in what we receive but in what we give and in the profound impact our love and compassion have on the lives of those we care for.

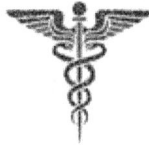

REFERENCES

1. Hippius, H., & Neundörfer, G. (2003). The discovery of Alzheimer's disease. *Dialogues in Clinical Neuroscience, 5*(1), 101–108. https://doi.org/10.31887/dcns.2003.5.1/hhippius

2. National Institute on Aging. (2017, May 16). *What Happens to the Brain in Alzheimer's Disease?* National Institute on Aging. https://www.nia.nih.gov/health/alzheimers-caues-and-risk-factors/what-happens-brain-alzheimers-disease

3. Assistant Secretary for Public Affairs (ASPA). (2023, December 12). *HHS Releases National Plan Update Marking Year of Progress on Alzheimer's Disease, Related Dementias.* U.S. Department of Health and Human Services. https://www.hhs.gov/about/news/2023/12/12/hhs-releases-national-plan-update-marking-year-of-progress-on-alzheimers-disease-related-dementias.html

4. Graff-Radford, J. (2022, June 11). *Alzheimer's and dementia: what's the difference?* Mayo Clinic. https://www.mayoclinic.org/es/diseases-conditions/alzheimers-disease/expert-answers/alzheimers-and-dementia-whats-the-difference/faq-20396861

5. WHO. (2023, March 15). *Dementia.* World Health Organization. https://www.who.int/news-room/fact-sheets/detail/dementia

6. Alzheimer's Society. (2015). *Signs of dementia seen 18 years before diagnosis | Alzheimer's Society.* Www.alzheimers.org.uk. https://www.alzheimers.org.uk/research/care-and-cure-research-magazine/signs-dementia-seen-18-years-diagnosis

7. Müller-Spahn, F. (2003). Behavioral disturbances in dementia. *Dialogues in Clinical Neuroscience, 5*(1), 49–59. https://doi.org/10.31887/DCNS.2003.5.1/fmuellerspahn

8. Alzheimer's Association. (2023). *Oral health and Alzheimer's risk.* Alzheimer's Disease and Dementia. https://www.alz.org/co/news/oral-health-and-alzheimers-risk

9. Fagan, A. M., Roe, C. M., Xiong, C., Mintun, M. A., Morris, J. C., & Holtzman, D. M. (2007). Cerebrospinal Fluid tau/β-Amyloid42 Ratio as a Prediction of Cognitive Decline in Nondemented Older Adults. *Archives of Neurology, 64*(3), 343–349. https://doi.org/10.1001/archneur.64.3.noc60123

10. Mayo Clinic Staff. (2019, April 19). *Diagnosing Alzheimer's: How Alzheimer's is diagnosed.* Mayo Clinic. https://www.mayoclinic.org/diseases-conditions/alzheimers-disease/in-depth/alzheimers/art-20048075

11. Freitas, S., Simões, M. R., Alves, L., & Santana, I. (2013). Montreal Cognitive Assessment: Validation Study for Mild Cognitive Impairment and Alzheimer Disease. *Alzheimer Disease & Associated Disorders, 27*(1), 37–43. https://doi.org/10.1097/wad.0b013e3182420bfe

12. Lai, N. M., Chang, S. M. W., Ng, S. S., Stanaway, F., Tan, S. L., & Chaiyakunapruk, N. (2019). Animal-assisted therapy for dementia. *Cochrane Database of Systematic Reviews, 2019*(1). https:// doi.org/10.1002/14651858.cd013243

13. Lam, H. L., Li, W. T. V., Laher, I., & Wong, R. Y. (2020). Effects of Music Therapy on Patients with Dementia—A Systematic Review. *Geriatrics, 5*(4), 62. https://doi.org/10.3390/geriatrics504 0062

14. Park, M., Song, R., Ju, K., Shin, J. C., Seo, J., Fan, X., Gao, X., Ryu, A., & Li, Y. (2023). Effects of Tai Chi and Qigong on cognitive and physical functions in older adults: system-

atic review, meta-analysis, and meta-regression of ran-
domized clinical trials. *BMC Geriatrics, 23*(1). https://doi.
org/10.1186/s12877-023-04070-2

15. Rahman, A., Hossen, M. A., Chowdhury, M. F. I., Bari, S., Taman-
na, N., Sultana, S. S., Haque, S. N., Al Masud, A., & Saif-Ur-
Rahman, K. M. (2023). Aducanumab for the treatment of
Alzheimer's disease: a systematic review. *Psychogeriatrics,
23*(3). https://doi.org/10.1111/psyg.12944

16. Commissioner, O. of the. (2023, January 6). *FDA Grants Accel-
erated Approval for Alzheimer's Disease Treatment.* FDA.
https://www.fda.gov/news-events/press-announcements/
fda-grants-accelerated-approval-alzheimers-disease-treat-
ment #:~:text=Today%2C%20the%20U.S.%20 Food%20and

17. Alzheimer's Association. (2023). *Alzheimer's disease facts and
figures. Alzheimer's Disease and Dementia*; Alzheimer's
Association. https://www.alz.org/alzheimers-dementia/
facts-figures

18. National Institute on Aging. (2023, March 1). *Alzheimer's Disease
Genetics Fact Sheet.* National Institute on Aging. https://
www.nia.nih.gov/health/genetics-and-family-history/alzhei-
mers-disease-genetics-fact-sheet

19. Johns Hopkins Medicine. (2013). *Blood Pressure and Alzheimer's Risk: What's the Connection?* John Hopkins
Medicine. https://www.hopkinsmedicine.org/health/con-
ditions-and-diseases/alzheimers-disease/blood-pressure-
and-alzheimers-risk-whats-the-connection

20. McDade, E., Bednar, M. M., Brashear, H. R., Miller, D. S., Maruff,
P., Randolph, C., Ismail, Z., Carrillo, M. C., Weber, C. J.,
Bain, L. J., & Hake, A. M. (2020). The pathway to secondary
prevention of Alzheimer's disease. *Alzheimer's &; Dementia: Translational Research &; Clinical Interventions, 6*(1).
https://doi.org/10.1002/trc2.12069

21. Alzheimer's Association. (2015). *Prevention.* Alzheimer's Disease and Dementia. https://www.alz.org/alzheimers-dementia/ research_progress/prevention

22. Sierra, C. (2020). Hypertension and the Risk of Dementia. *Frontiers in Cardiovascular Medicine, 7*(5). https://doi. org/10.3389/fcvm.2020.00005

23. Spira, A. P., Chen-Edinboro, L. P., Wu, M. N., & Yaffe, K. (2014). Impact of sleep on the risk of cognitive decline and dementia. *Current Opinion in Psychiatry, 27*(6), 478–483. https:// doi.org/10.1097/yco.0000000000000106

24. Gracia-García, P., Bueno-Notivol, J., Lipnicki, D. M., de la Cámara, C., Lobo, A., & Santabárbara, J. (2023). Clinically significant anxiety as a risk factor for Alzheimer's disease: Results from a 10-year follow-up community study. *International Journal of Methods in Psychiatric Research, 32*(3). https://doi.org/10.1002/mpr.1934

25. Huang, A. R., Roth, D. L., Cidav, T., Chung, S., Amjad, H., Thorpe, R. J., Boyd, C. M., & Cudjoe, T. K. M. (2023). Social isolation and 9-year dementia risk in community-dwelling Medicare beneficiaries in the United States. *Journal of the American Geriatrics Society, 71*(3). https://doi.org/10.1111/jgs.18140

26. CDC. (2023, July 13). *About Alzheimer's Disease | Aging.* www.cdc.gov. https://www.cdc.gov/aging/alzheimers-disease-dementia/about-alzheimers.html

27. Alzheimer's Association. (2021). 2021 Alzheimer's disease facts and figures. *Alzheimer's & Dementia, 17*(3). https://doi.org/10.1002/alz.12328

28. Alzheimer's Association. (2020). 2020 Alzheimer's Disease Facts and Figures. *Alzheimer's & Dementia, 16*(3), 391–460. https://doi.org/10.1002/alz.12068

29. Alzheimer's Association. (2022). *Hispanic Americans More Likely to Develop Dementia. Why?*Alzheimer's Disease and Dementia. https://www.alz.org/news/2022/hispanic-americans-more-likely-to-develop-dementia#:~:text=Hispanic%20Americans%20are%201.5%20times

30. Alzheimer's Association. (2020). *Primary Care Physicians on the Front Lines of Diagnosing and Providing Alzheimer's and Dementia Care.* Alzheimer's Disease and Dementia. https://www.alz.org/news/2020/primary-care-physicians-on-the-front-lines-of-diag#:~:text=The%20report%20found%20that%2082

31. Stefanacci, R. G. (2011). The costs of Alzheimer's disease and the value of effective therapies. *The American Journal of Managed Care, 17 Suppl 13*, S356-362. https://pubmed.ncbi.nlm.nih.gov/22214393/#:~:text=Every%2069%20seconds%2C%20a%20person

32. UsAgainstAlzheimer's. (2023, November 21). *Alzheimer's Disease: Get The Facts.* UsAgainstAlzheimer's. https://www.usagainstalzheimers.org/alzheimers-disease-get-facts#:~:text=Alzheimer%27s%20Affects%20Millions&text=The%20number%20of%20Americans%20with

33. Alzheimer's Association. (2019). *New Alzheimer's Association Report Shows Significant Disconnect Between Seniors, Physicians When.* Alzheimer's Disease and Dementia. https://www.alz.org/news/2019/new-alzheimer-s-association-report-shows-signifi

34. Lang, L., Clifford, A., Wei, L., Zhang, D., Leung, D., Augustine, G., Danat, I. M., Zhou, W., Copeland, J. R., Anstey, K. J., & Chen, R. (2017). Prevalence and determinants of undetected dementia in the community: a systematic literature review and a meta-analysis. BMJ *Open, 7*(2), e011146. https://doi.org/10.1136/bmjopen-2016-011146

35. Eiser, A. R. (2017). Why does Finland have the highest dementia mortality rate? Environmental factors may be generalizable. *Brain Research, 1671*, 14–17. https://doi.org/10.1016/j.brainres.2017.06.032

36. Alzheimer's Association. (2023). *Stages of Alzheimer's.* Alzheimer's Disease and Dementia; Alzheimer's Association. https://www.alz.org/alzheimers-dementia/stages

37. Salamon, M. (2023, February 1). *Managing the unthinkable.* Harvard Health. https://www.health.harvard.edu/mind-and-mood/managing-the-unthinkable

38. Cintra, M. T. G., de Rezende, N. A., de Moraes, E. N., Cunha, L. C. M., & da Gama Torres, H. O. (2014). A comparison of survival, pneumonia, and hospitalization in patients with advanced dementia and dysphagia receiving either oral or enteral nutrition. *The Journal of Nutrition, Health and Aging, 18*(10), 894–899. https://doi.org/10.1007/s12603-014-0487-3

39. National Institute on Aging. (2022, November 17). *Providing Care and Comfort at the End of Life.* National Institute on Aging. https://www.nia.nih.gov/health/end-life/providing-care-and-comfort-end-life

40. National Institute on Aging. (2021, May 14). *What Are Palliative Care and Hospice Care?* National Institute on Aging. https://www.nia.nih.gov/health/hospice-and-palliative-care/what-are-palliative-care-and-hospice-care

41. Li, I. (2002). Feeding Tubes in Patients with Severe Dementia. *American Family Physician, 65*(8), 1605–1611. https://www.aafp.org/pubs/afp/issues/2002/0415/p1605.html

42. World Health Organization. (2023, March 31). *Depressive Disorder (depression).* World Health Organization. https://www.who.int/news-room/fact-sheets/detail/depression

43. Alves, L. C. de S., Monteiro, D. Q., Bento, S. R., Hayashi, V. D., Pelegrini, L. N. de C., & Vale, F. A. C. (2019). Burnout syndrome in informal caregivers of older adults with dementia: A systematic review. *Dementia & Neuropsychologia, 13*(4), 415–421. https://doi.org/10.1590/1980-57642018dn13-040008

44. Alfakhri, A. S., Alshudukhi, A. W., Alqahtani, A. A., Alhumaid, A. M., Alhathlol, O. A., Almojali, A. I., Alotaibi, M. A., & Alaqeel, M. K. (2018). Depression Among Caregivers of Patients With Dementia. INQUIRY: *The Journal of Health Care Organization, Provision, and Financing, 55*, 004695801775043. https://doi.org/10.1177/0046958017750432

45. Alzheimers.gov. (2023). *Tips for Caregivers and Families of People With Dementia.* National Institute on Aging. https://www.alzheimers.gov/life-with-dementia/tips-caregivers

46. Hanson, L. C., Ersek, M., Gilliam, R., & Carey, T. S. (2011). Oral feeding options for people with dementia: A systematic review. *Journal of the American Geriatrics Society, 59*(3), 463–472. https://doi.org/10.1111/j.1532-5415.2011.03320.x

47. Warden, V., Hurley, A. C., & Volicer, L. (2003). *Pain Assessment IN Advanced Dementia (PAINAD).* https://www.hhs.texas.gov/sites/default/files/documents/doing-business-with-hhs/provider-portal/QMP/painad.pdf

48. Kato-Narita, E. M., & Radanovic, M. (2009). Characteristics of falls in mild and moderate Alzheimer's disease. *Dementia & Neuropsychologia, 3*(4), 337–343. https://doi.org/10.1590/s1980-57642009dn30400013

49. Derouesné, C., Guigot, J., Chermat, V., Winchester, N., & Lacomblez, L. (1996). Sexual Behavioral Changes in Alzheimer Disease. *Alzheimer Disease & Associated Disorders, 10*(2), 86. https://doi.org/10.1007/s11940-016-0425-2

50. Alzheimer's Society. (2019). *Toilet problems and continence.* Alzheimer's Society. https://www.alzheimers.org.uk/get-support/daily-living/toilet-problems-continence

51. Savory, G. (2017, April 6). *Alzheimer's Disease And Incontinence.* Bladder & Bowel Community. https://www.bladderandbowel.org/associated-illness/alzheimers-and-incontinence/

52. Johns Hopkins Medicine. (2019). *Bedsores.* Johns Hopkins Medicine. https://www.hopkinsmedicine.org/health/condtions-and-diseases/bedsores

53. Evans, A. (2019). *What is Communication? - Definition & Importance - Video & Lesson Transcript | Study.com.* Study.com. https://study.com/academy/lesson/what-is-communication-definition-importance.html

54. National Institute on Aging. (n.d.). *Managing Money Problems for People With Dementia.* National Institute on Aging. https://www.nia.nih.gov/health/legal-and-financial-planning/managing-money-problems-people-dementia

55. Family Caregiver Alliance. (n.d.). *The Sandwich Generation: When Caregiver Seems to Be Your Only Role.* Family Caregiver Alliance. https://www.caregiver.org/news/sandwich-generation-when-caregiver-seems-be-your-only-role/

ABOUT THE AUTHOR

Dr. Annette Acevedo Hernandez, MD, CDS

Dr. Annette Acevedo Hernandez is a distinguished physician and dementia care specialist with over 25 years of experience in the field. As the author of *Alzheimer's & Other Dementias: A Caregiver's Guide,* she draws upon her extensive expertise to offer invaluable insights and practical advice for caregivers. Dr. Acevedo Hernandez has served as a primary care physician and medical director of a nursing home for over 25 years, where she has dedicated herself to the care and well-being of patients with Alzheimer's and other dementias.

Her passion for dementia care is deeply rooted in personal experience, as she embarked on this journey over two decades ago when her father was diagnosed with Alzheimer's. Inspired by her caregiving journey, Dr. Annette Acevedo Hernandez has devoted her career to various roles encompassing prevention, diagnosis, and treatment. She intimately understands the challenges caregivers face, especially during the late stages of the disease, and is committed to providing unwavering support and guidance.

Dr. Acevedo Hernandez's mission is to enhance the quality of life for individuals affected by Alzheimer's and other dementias through comprehensive care and support. To learn more about Dr. Annette Acevedo Hernandez and her work, please visit her website at www.DementiaCareMD.com.

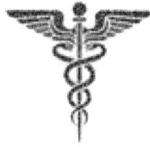

ABOUT THE COLLABORATOR

Dr. Gilfredy Acevedo Hernandez, MD

Dr. Gilfredy Acevedo Hernandez brings over 30 years of expertise as an internal medicine and medical acupuncture physician to his role as a collaborator for the nonfiction book *Alzheimer's & Other Dementias: A Caregiver's Guide.*

His passion for enhancing the quality of life for individuals with Alzheimer's and dementia ignited 25 years ago when his father was diagnosed with Alzheimer's disease. Having witnessed firsthand the impact the condition had on his family and having served as both a primary care physician and a consulting MD at a nursing home for more than 20 years. Dr. Acevedo partnered with his sister Dr. Annette Acevedo Hernandez, as a collaborator to share both his personal and clinical journey as a caregiver. His primary objective is to spearhead a mission aimed at making a meaningful difference in the lives of patients and caregivers alike. His dedication to raising awareness and fostering compassionate care underscores his invaluable contribution to this indispensable resource for caregivers.

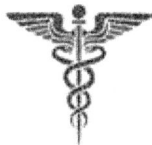

ABOUT THE TRANSLATOR

Camille A. Schwinghammer, MSMS

Camille A. Schwinghammer serves as the translator for *Alzheimer's & Other Dementias: A Caregiver's Guide.* Committed to ensuring the widespread accessibility of this invaluable resource, Schwinghammer's expertise is rooted in her academic background and practical experience. Holding a Bachelor's in Clinical Psychology from the University of Central Florida and a Master's in Medical Science from Jacksonville University, she seamlessly combines academic rigor with real-world insight in her translation work. Her dedication to accuracy and attention to detail are evident in her meticulous translations, underscoring her vital role in making this guide accessible to readers worldwide.